SURGERY IN AYURVEDA

(Shalya Shalakya)

Indian Medical Science Series No. 137

SURGERY IN AYURVEDA

(Shalya Shalakya)

Edited by

Prof. Dr. P.H. Kulkarni

Sri Satguru Publications

A Division of

Indian Books Centre
Delhi, India

Published by
Sri Satguru Publications,
Indological and Oriental Publishers
A Division of
Indian Books Centre
40/5, Shakti Nagar,
Delhi-110007
India

First Edition; Delhi , 2008

ISBN 81-7030-898-4

Printed at Sachin Printers, Delhi

Dedicated to
Students and
Research workers
in the field of
Surgery (Shalya-Shalakya)
—Prof. P. H. Kulkarni
Sydney
Australia
April 2006

Contents

Few words :

I was much interested in Surgery during my student days. After graduation I worked in minor surgery department of Hospital and after wards worked as assistant to Dr. H. N. Phadnis in gynaecological operations for five years in his Hospital.

During last three decades we organised many professional development programmes, Training programme for overseas Students & International Conferences workshops in India & abroad. Various topics related to surgical procedures in all these events.

This book is a complilation of many articles, lectures, papers related to surgery i.e. Shalya Shalakya. I am grateful to all contributors, authors, who participated in all these Ayurvedic Seminars. This is compilation of all such research oriented papers in the field of Surgery in Ayurveda during last half century. Lord Dhanvantaree bless every body!

—Prof. P. H. Kulkarni

Chapter 1
Shalya

—Dr. S. I. Nagral

Ayurveda popularly known as Ashtang Ayurveda, is the science of life comprising of Shalya, Shalakya, Kaychikitsa, Kaumarbhritya, Agadtantra, Bhootvidya, Rasayana and Vajikaran. It is the science in which the knowledge of life exists and which promotes longevity. Though considered a sub-division of Atharva veda, the present day Ayurveda is based upon the individual experiences in the realm of cure and prevention, collected from various sources and documented in the form of Samhitas etc. The dual object of Ayurveda are promotion and maintenance of health in the healthy and alleviation of the disease in the afflicted. The medical man from the eternity has always been trying to prevent old age, to relieve pain, to ally fear and to conquer death.

Shalya tantra is the first, foremost and important branch of Ayurveda. Shalya as a source for the suffering in the human body could be internal like the deranged doshas or external like foreign bodies entering the body. The detailed study of the consequences of Shalya and their management including the methods of removal forms is the scope of this branch. Sushrut describes as —

Vividh Truna Kashtha Pashanapanshu Loha Asthi Balnakha

Pooyastrave Antargarbha Shalyoddharnartham Yantra

Shastra Ksharagni Pranidhan Vrana Vinishchayartham/

Wherein various extraneous substances like hay, wooden - splinters, stone fragments etc. enter the body and the deranged body fluids like pus and the obstructive foetus be have as Shalya - studying their effects and devising methods for the removal of the same, as well as the rational utility of instruments, Caustics and Cautery for multiple purposes, diagnosis & management of wounds constitute Shalyatantra.

Generally the study of the conditions amenable to manipulative procedures with the aid of surgical instruments is considered as Shalyachikitsa.

Sushrut is one of the outstanding luminaries of Indian medicine. He was emphatically a surgeon and a renowned author and editor. Sushrut Samhita, the only exhaustive book available today, deals with the problems mainly concerned with Shalya tantra. Though number of other Samhitas of the contemporaries of Sushruta like Aurabhra, Aupadhenav etc. are mentioned, none are available. The documentation as it stands, narrates not only the detailed description of the surgical diseases existed then but also can contribute a great lot to the management of surgical conditions prevalent today. Sushrut has always considered the study of Shalya tantra as supreme and assigned highest value, because of the elaborate parapharnelia used, description of the other tantras here and the methods of treatment being quick and remunerative.

Being unable to trace the origin of science of life, the scientists of today are compelled to attribute the same to Brahma. It is accepted that Brahma created the world and created the science of life too. The following table explains in nutshell the evolution :-

Brahma

Prajapathi

Ashvinikumaras

Indra

- Atreya Sampradaya (School of Medicine)
- Kashyapa Sampradaya (School of OB-GYN and Paediatrics)
- Dhanvantari Sampradaya (School of surgery) Sushruta
  - Shalya (General Surgery)
  - Shalakya (ENT, Opthalmology, Craniology
  - Kayachikitsa (General Medicine)
  - Kaumar Bhritya (Obst., Gyanaecology & Paediatrics)
  - Agad tantra (Toxicology)
  - Bhoot Vidya (Demonology)
  - Rasayan (Rejuvenation)
  - Vaji karan (Aphrodisiacs)

Ethical standards then were very high. Surgical ethics was well-defined.

"No other gift is better than the gift of life" was considered as one of the high ideals of medical profession.

"He who treats his patients only on humanitarian grounds without desiring any financial or personal gains supersedes all other physicians and those who trade their medical skills for mere livelihood can be considered as collecting a pile of dust leaving aside a heap of real gold.

And also he who regards kindness to humanity as his supreme religion and treats his patients accordingly succeeds in fulfilling his ambition of life and derives pleasure."

The fact that the patient may doubt his relatives; his sons and even his parents, but he has full faith in his doctor and submits himself to his care, without any misgivings, proves that the doctor has to behave in a befitting manner. Hence if he is preached - "Always pray for the well being of all creatures. Fullest efforts should be tried to cure the sick throughout day and night, however you may be engaged. Have no ill-fellings towards the patients even for the sake of your living or life. You should not commit adultery even in thought, nor covet others possessions. Try to be simple and modest in your dress as well as in appearance. Do not be a drunkard. Neither do a sin nor associate your-self with any sinner. Your language should be gentle, pure righteous, courteous, worthy, true, wholesome and moderate. You should take your past exprience into account. Always try to increase your knowledge and equipment. Don't boast too much of your knowledge, even though you may possess it. Others get offended by the boastfulness of even capable persons.

Practice could be started only after having read and thoroughly studied the medical science, having seen and performed operations himself, having passed the essential tests and then obtained the permission of the Governing Authority. Registration was compulsory before anyone embarked on medical practice.

As said by Sushruta, "he who knows theory only, he is not good at practical work gets bewildered on being confronted with a patient in the same way a coward feels on the battle-field. On the otherhand, he who is good in practical work because of his boldness, but lacks in theory, he is not respected by Pundits. In fact, he deserves punishment by the State. Both these types of persons can not be considered as experts and are not capable to work properly. They possess one-sided knowledge and can be compared to birds with one wing. Hence only the prudents having theoretical background and the practical experience are capable to succeed as two wheeled vehicles are useful in the battle field."

A surgeon was expected to have boldness, swiftness, sharpness of instruments, no sweating, steady hands and confidence.

In his apparel, he was expected to wear white and sober dress, keep his hairs short and clip the nails and attend to personal hygiene and cleanliness.

On his visits he should go with a cool balanced mind, wishing everybody without trying to show off, with an attitude to help and accompanied by an able assistant. He was cautioned about his behaviour towards the members of the family of the patients, specially the ladies.

In order to broaden his knowledge and outlook, he was expected to study the subject regularly and take part in scientific debates and discussions, observe the allied sciences and take training from specialists of those branches.

Sushruta always considered "the person who studied one branch of science only cannot arrive at proper conclusions, the physician, therefore, should learn as many related sciences as possible."

Academically the physician was expected to be fullfledged following the instructions, self-assessment and rationalising the treatment as per the necessity in management of cases.

Experimental surgery, management of emergencies, dealing with the dieing and the dead were also the topics discussed in ethical management. Quacks and quackery were highly condemned.

It was compulsory for a student to undergo practical training in operative surgery. The basic procedures like excision and incision etc. were practised on various substances and then only he was allowed to assist regular operations on human beings. Subsequently he was allowed to operate, himself with the assistance and under the supervision on the seniors. After completion of this course, the candidate was allowed to register and start medical practice.

The practical procedure of excision was practised on Alabu, water melon and cucumber.

The art of taking incision and extending the same as per necessity was taught by making an opening in the body of a lather bag full of water.

Scrapping was taught on a piece of skin on which the hair is allowed to remain.

Venesection was taught on the vein of a dead animal or on the lotus stem.

The art of probing was taught on the worm-eating wood. The extraction was taught by practising the art of withdrawing the seeds from a jack fruit or by achieving extraction of the teeth from the jaw of a dead animal.

The process of evacuation was taught on the surface of a shalmali plant covered with a coat of wax.

The art of suturing was taught on pieces of cloth, skin or hyde.

Similarly the art of bandaging could practically be learant by bandaging a full size model, whereas the art of reconstructing the ear lobules should be practically demonstrated on a soft severed muscle.

The art of cauterisation and applying caustics should

be demonstrated on a piece of soft flesh and lastly the art of inserting syringes, administering enema in the region of bladder or in a wound should be taught by asking the pupil to insert a tube into the lateral fissure of a pitcher, full of water or in the mouth of gourd.

[Reference : Intensive Training Programme for Australian Students 1988]

Chapter 2

Practice of Surgery

SHALYA 2

—Dr. S. I. Nagral

Instruments used for various purposes in surgery were mainly classified as surgical appliances (blunt instruments) and sharp cutting instruments. The former mainly were utilised for different devices and the latter for regular operative procedures.

Surgical appliance or yantras were accounted as 101 in number and were grouped as per the functional utility.

1.	Swastika (Forceps)	24
2.	Sandansha (Tongs)	2
3.	Talayantra	2
4.	Nadiyantra (Tubular)	20
5.	Shalakas (probes)	28
6.	Upayantras	25

These instruments were all made of iron/steel which may be stubstituted for any other similar or suitable substance, where iron could not be available. The terminal ends of these appliances are usually made to resemble those of birds or beasts. Hence they looked like some animal beaks. They were all devised on the advice of an experienced surgeon and according to the directions laid down in the medical text of recognised authority or according to the exigencies of the case as per the same and structure of other appliances used on similar occasions.

The yantras should be made neither too large nor too small, and their edges should be sharp with a special eye to strengthen and keep steady by providing a convenient handle.

These Swastik yantras should be made to measure 18 fingers in length, and their mouths should be made to resemble those of lions, tigers wolves, bears, cats, jackle etc. The two halves of the yantra should be weled together by means of a bolt resembling a masura pulse (lential) in size and the handle should be turned inwards in the shape of a mace or Ankusha. Such appliances can be used in extracting any thorn or a foregin material which may have entered into the bones. Sandansha yantras could be with a catch or without they should be made to measure 16 fingers in length and are used to take out any thorn-like substance from the subcutaneous areas, muscle, vein or nerves.

The Talayantras which measure 12 fingers in length were classified as single and the double Talaya. They are used for removing the foreign bodies from the nose, ears and other external channels or passages of the body.

The Nadiyantras like syrinches, with a passage or an aperture running throughtheir entire length are constructd in a variety of shapes, sizes and for multiple purposes. The length and the circumference should be made to commonsurate with those of the passage of human system intended to be introduced. For example, the ones needed for fistula, phimosis, ascites uretheral conditions etc.

The Shalakas are of different size and shape. The circumference and the length is needed to be adjusted as per the individual necessity like the ones for measuring the length of a track, the other one for detecting the substance into a cavity etc. Depending upon the shape, they are named as Sharapunkha, Sarpaphalakariti Gandoopada etc.

The Upayantras Viz. the minor surgical accessories include substances like silk thread, bark creeper, linen, stones hammer etc.

The functions of these yantras are :

1. Nirghatan - Withdrawing a shalya by moving to and fro.
2. Pooran - Filling and pouring drugs in cavities.
3. Bandhan - Bandaging
4. Vyuvan - Cutting and withdrawing a shalya.
5. Vartan - Resetting by means of a twirling motion.
6. Chalan - Moving a shalya from one place to another.
7. Vivartan - Twisting
8. Vivaran - Expanding
9. Peedan - Pressing
10. Margavishodan - Purifying the passage.
11. Vikarsan - Drawing off
12. Aharan - Extracting
13. Anchan - Bringing to the surface
14. Punnaman - Lifting
15. Vinaman - Lowering
16. Bhanjan - Applying pressure all raround on a part.
17. Unmathan - Agitating
18. Achushan - Sucking
19. Ashan - Probing

20. Daran - Cleaving
21. Rujukaran - Straightening
22. Prakshalan - Flushing
23. Pradhaman - Stuffing the nose
24. Pramarjan - Cleaning

The sharp cutting instruments or Shastras are twenty in number as –

Mandalagra	-	six fingers in length & is provided with round or circular face.
Karapatra	-	Saw
Vridhipatra	-	Surgical knife measuring seven fingers in length.
Nakhashastra	-	Nail clipper measuring four fingers in length of the blade.
Mudrika	-	Ring with a blade
Utpalapatra	-	Resembles a lotus leaf in shape.
Ardhadhara	-	Lancet measuring eight fingers in length.
Suchi	-	Suture needle.
Kushapatra	-	Shaped like the blade of a Kusha grass.
Atemukha	-	resembling the bill of a bird of Ate species, measuring seven fingers in length.
Shararimukh	-	Scissors measuring twelve fingers in length.
Antarmukh	-	Semicircular in shape.
Trikurchak	-	Trocar with three blades measuring eight fingers in length.
Kutharika	-	Blunt axe (Gum elevator)

Vrihimukh - Trocar measuring six fingers in length.

Ara - resembles the awl of a cobbler measuring ten fingers in length.

Vetaspatra - Knife measuring eight fingers in length.

Vadisha - Hook

Dantashanku - Pincers for extracting tooth.

Eshani - Probe

These instruments are fitted with handles of easy grip and are made of good & pure iron well shaped, sharp, and are set with edges that are not jagged and end in well formed points or tops, should be deemed as the best of their kind.

The edges were tempered by an alkali, water or oil. For instruments used for cutting an arrow, a bone or a penetrating shalya the edges were tempered by alkali, those used for cleaving cutting muscle water was used and for siravedh and snayuchhedan oil was used.

The Anushastras are the skin of bamboos, Crytals, Bits of glass, Fire, Nails etc.

The basic operative procedures are –

Chhedan - is undertaken in Bhagandara, Shlaishak Granthi, Tilakalaka, Arbuda, Arsha, Charmakila, Jatumani, Mansa sangatha, Galashundi, Valmika, Vranavatma, Shatponaka,
Adhrusa, Upadansha, Mansakandi as well as shalyas.

Bhedan - Vidradhi, Pakwashotha, Talu puppata, Dantapuppata etc.

Lekhan - Rohinis, Kilas, Upajiva, Danta vaidarbha, Granthi, Vranavartma, etc.

Vedhana - Dakodara, Mutravridhi etc.

Aharya - Dantasharkara, Shalya etc.

Visravan - Vidradhi, Kushta, Visarpa etc.

Seevan - could be undertaken in clean and traumatic wounds, The types of stitching like Anuvellita, Rujugranthi, Gophanika and Tunnasevani are used depending upon the type of the condition.

The combination of these basic operative procedures can be utilised to design a specific operation for a disease.

[Reference : Intensive Training Programme for Australian Students 1988]

Chapter 3

Utpatti (origin)

Period of Ruk-sanhita or Rugwed-sanhita is–4000 years B.C.

Period of Taitiriya Sanhita–3000 years B.C. References are found stating surgical procedures like correction of dislocated shoulder, leg lost in war replaced by Iron prosthesis.

Later on - Period of Atharbvasamhita, a period of development of Shalyatantra. Hence we find references stating :

1) Catheterisation for retention of urine.

2) Suregical procedurers performed on urinary system like removal of a bladder calculus..

3) Caeserine section for obstructed labour.

Shalya-tantra received a little setback during Buddha period, i.e. years 250 B.C. to years 300 A.C.

Sushrut-sanhita the basic important ancient text related to shalya-tantra was written between period years 600 to years 500 B.C.

Before Sushrut-samhita literature relarted to surgical practice were many, like written by Bhoj, Aushadhanev, Aurabhra, Vaitaran, Pushkalvat, Nimi. Their original work is not available now. Sushruta has referred these in his text. Sushrut-sanhita presently available was published by Nagarjuna in first century.

Sushrut-sanhita was translated in Arabic language by MANKH in 9th century, says- Abdul Faraz - an Arabic writer.

SHALYAS TANTRA - SUSHRUT SANHITA deals with following surgical conditions :

Vranashotha (Inflammations)

vrana (Ulcers and wounds)

Vidradhis (Abscesses - superficial and deep)

Nadivrana and Bhagander (Sinuses and fistuae)

Vat-vyadhi (esp. Vatarakta - Gangrenes because of blood vascular diseases)

Grudhrasi (Sciatica)

Ardit (Fascial paraysis)

Pakshaghat (Hemiplegia)

Apatantrak (Tetanus)

Arsha (Piles - haemdrrhoids)

Ashmari (Urinary Calculus)

Kushtha (Surgical conditions related to skin)

Prameh (Diabetes mallitus)

Udar (Ascitis)

Moodhagarbha ( )

Stanarog (Diseases related to breast)

Visarpa (Cellulitis)

Ganda-mala-Apachi (Tuberculous lymphadenitis and cold abscesses)

Galaganda (Goitre)

Vruddhi (Hernia - Hydrocele)

Upadansha (Vineral diseases)

Shleepada (Elephantasis)

Bhagna (Fractures)

Diseases related to oral cavity, lips, teeth, palate, throat

Shalya tantra also deals with embryology and development of the foetus, vast description of different blood vessels and lymphatic vessels in the body - Marmas (Vital points in the body) muscles, bones and joints, different methods of Surgical practice, different surgical instruments used in surgery Ksharkarma (Alkaine Cantom) Agnikarma (cauterization and its applications) Raktamokshan (blood letting and its application Vranalepan vidhi (Application of different medicated pastes) Splints and bandages. Detail description of Panchakarma treatment and its application in surgical diseases.

Valuable description of different food materials like milk and milk products, edible oils, honey, sugarcane, medicated wines, urines of different animals and their medicinal properites in surgical diseases.

Meat of different animals, fruits, vegetables, flowers, roots, different salts, different useful metals, pearls, diamonds, corals, rules and regulations about diet and their role in treating different diseases are also included in Shalyatantra.

Shalyatantra (Sushruta) in its Dravyasangrahaniya chapter describes innumerbale herbal medicines for different surgical as well as medical diseases.

From all this treasure from Shalyatantra one can find definate solutions for many difficult or incurable disease conditions and can help smooth recovery in many other diseases.

VRANASHOTHA

Inflammatory swelling, locaised elevated, even or uneven in size but noncystic, related to Twacha (skin) and Mansa (Soft-tissues).

There are three stages

1. Amavastha (Early inflammatory stage) - When swelling is firm, with less amount of pain - swelling i.e. oedema is less, colour of the overlying skin is not changed much, - low fever.

2. Pachhamanavastha - (Acute inflammatory stage) There are three types of pains like pricking, cutting, like stings of the ants, burning giving rise to restlessness. Swelling is more, overlying skin is stretched and its colour is also changed. There is fever, thirst, loss of appetite.

Pakwa-vastha - (Ripe stage) pains are reduced, swelling decreases. Overllying skin becomes pale and wrinkled, skin starts peeling off, there is fluctuation. In between there is a pain and itching, fever and thirst decreases. Appetite starts improving.

Types :

1. Vataja - Black coloured swelling, soft with rough skin, pains waxing and wanning.
2. Pittaja - Yellow or red in colour, soft, rapidly spreading and with burning pains.
3. Kaphaj - White, hard, slowly progressing with heaviness, itching.
4. Tridoshaj - All above symptoms & signs
5. Raktaj - like pitta type but more black in colour.
6. Agantu - (Because of external assaults) like pittaj and raktaj, iron like in colour.

First 5 types occur because of Samprapti (Pathology) taking place inside the body.

In case of a Kaphaj and traumatic type it is difficult to assess whether it is unripe or ripe. In that case flactuation is the important sign.

It is very necessary for a doctor to know all the three stages to trerat the patient in time and to save his life. He who does not know this is called thief (Taskar).

TREATMENT

Procedures followed are as under:

1. Vimlapan - Meaning of the word is massaging the swelling with the help of fingres but it is not desired. This should consist of.

   Lepa - Application of medicated paste on the swelling (pastes of different thickness).

   Parishek - To pour decoctions or medicated oils on the swelling.

   Abhyang - Application of oil to the body.

   Swed - Application of steam.

   These procedures are followed to limit it and to reverse it (to help the defence mechanism of the body).

   Internal administration of different appropriate medicines (Shaman Chikitsa) is also included.

2. Avasechan - Blood letting, - Emesis, (Vaman) purgation (Virechana)

3. Upanah - Application of different medicated pastes on the swelling.

   Above three procedures are used in first two stages viz. Amavastha and Pacchamanavastha.

   Blood letting (Raktamokshan) is described as very useful method in the treatment :

4. Bhedan - (Incision & drainage) ➔ of course to take adequate large cruciate incision.

5. Shodhan - To remove the remaining discharges and debris with the help of decoctions, medicated oils etc.

6. Ropan - To help the healing of the wound.

   Vaikrutapah - To take care of the healing and

healed wound and skin above if some deformities occur.

Sookshma triphala, Gandhak Rasayan, Sookshma Chaturbhuj of Ayurveda Rasashala, Pune are the best medicines for internal administration.

Atasi Upanah or Lepagoli for external application.

If incision is taken in Amavastha, bleeding occurs more. Pains are more, the pathology spreads, goes deep down and involves deeper structures and causes sever damage. This also can result into sinus and fistule formation i.e. (Nadivran).

Pathyapathya

Heavy to digest - sour and irritating and hygroscopic type of food is avoided. After incision and drainage Sansarjan is to be followed strictly.

Chapter 4
Vidradhi (Abscess)

Process of suppuration occurs early therefore called as. Vidradhi.

Violation of food regime, intake of stale food, too much of Alcohol consumption, excessive physical fatigue, intake of heavy indigestive food materials in excess and external trauma are the causes of Vidradhi.

It involves skin, blood, soft, tissues, fatty tissue, muscles, tendons and even bones causing serious swelling.

Main Types - Bahya (External) Abhyantar (Deep seated)

Types of Bahya-Vidradhi

Any fistulous communication throwing urine and other irritating discharges inferfer with healing.

The ulcers in patients suffering from diabetes, spinal cord diseases resulting into paralysis, distal obstructive conditions in different tracts, cellutitis, osteomylitis and ulcers with magets formation are very difficult to cure.

INCURABLE ULCER (Asadhya Vran)

Ulcer with excessive overgrowth of granulation tissue in its floor, discharging pus trapped inside, elevated apperence like that of vagina of mare thickened everted hornt excresences, from ulcer, elevated in the centre or deep cavity in the centre, with dirty and abnormal discharges like faces, urine, C.S.F. are said to be incurable.

Ulcers in patients with lot of spreading cellulitis, blisters formations fever, diarrehoea, severe thirst (dehydration) cough, breathlessness, restlessness, sleeplessness are said to be incurable.

Sushrut - has said that if not treated properly curable ulcers become difficult to cure and difficult become incurable.

BAD SIGNS

Any abnormality in respect of smell, colour, noies, touch and shape occuring in ulcer.

If there is a good a smell of wine, ghee, lower, louts, sandle, CHAMPAK flower or bad smell like the purulent dry flesh of a Dog. Horse, rat, crwo or smell like that of bedbug. Wet-soil or soil, they are bad signs.

In case of Pittaj Vran a colour like safforn, black colour or KANKUSHTA if seen and there is no burning pain, it is a bad sign.

In Kaphaj Vran severpain and burning.

Vran at vital pont with black thin discharge is a bad sign.

Ulcer with gas formation and abnormal noises, appearing like red hot fire is a bad sign. If shape of the ulcer is like a flag, chariot, worm, palace SHAKTI (Type of weapon) is a bad sign.

Cold feel from outside but severe burning pain inside and vice-versa is a bad sign.

In Spite of Proper treatment if there is no progress it should be considered as incurable ulcer.

Examination of Vran

1. Darshan - Inspection

Age of the patient colour of the wound and discharge, body and different organs, swelling, oedema etc. are inspected.

2. Prashna - Questions asked

   1. Vataja - Blackish colored rogh, severe pains, fainting
   2. Kukshi - In the join
   3. Vankshan - Appeared icular abscess side.
   4. Vrukka - Related to kidney - Perinephric abscess
   5. Vakrul - Live abscess
   6. Pleeha - Related to spleen
   7. Hriday - Related to heart may be pericarlial effusin or brain abscess
   8. Kloma - Pancreatic abscess

In all deep seated Vidradis (abscession pains at respective sties are severe with high fever perspiration, hasee, sometimes vomitting, constipation and toxic condition in the blood). One more type described is only related to women occuring after abortin or parturition related to female genital organs in the petric cavity.

Principles of treatment

Upanah

Swedan

Raktamokshan (Blood letting)

When ripe - incision (drainage)

Shodhan

Ropen

Chapter 5

Vrana (Ulcer)

One which is caused by pathology taking place in certain area of the body with change in colour of the skin above and without descrucion of the tissues affected though it heals, leaves a permanent scar behind is called Vrana.

Types

Nij (Because of indigenous causes) - 15 sub types depending upon predominence of Dosha)

Agantu (Because of external trauma of any form) -

1. Ghrushta - abrasion - loss of skin

2. Chhinna - incised wound

3. Bhinna - the injury or wound which occurs because of sharp pointed object or weapon reaching hollow viscus in the body and therefore of serious type.

4. Viddha - occuring because of sharp weapon deep but not involving a viscus.

5. Kshat - which is deep in centre and has signs of Chinna and Bhinna types.

6. Picchit - crushed injury. The tissues are compressed with or without external injury on the skin.

Clinical picture in Nij Vrana will depend upon the predominence of Dosha responsible. Vataja Vran - looking blackish, black or ash coloured or bone coloured, cold, dry-hard, not spreading much involved tissue is less, discharge like meatwash or curds water, little slimy and less in quantity Stretching type of pain.

Pittaj Vran - develops very soon, yellow, blue, orange coloured, burning pain. Tending towards suppuration very fast, lot of thirst, fever, prepiration discharge is reddish, oily, hot, more in quantity and foul smelling, sometimes purulent discharge.

Kaphaj Vran - White in colour, much itching sensation, less pain, thick edges, blood vessels and muscle fibres are seen in it and discharge from ulcer is cold, oily, white, slimy thick.

Raktaja Vran - looks like collection of corals, blackish, blisters arond it, smelling like strong kshar i.e. strong alkali (smell like that present in horse' residence) bloodly discharge, purulent discharge as if fumes coming from it.

Vatapittaj - burning, fuming.

Vatakaphaj - heaviness, itching, slimy little discharge.

Vataraktaja - dry, medium thick ulcer, little pains with less sensation, black sangouinous discharge.

Pittaraktag - fishwater like smell, soft, spreading, hot, blackish discharge.

Kapharaktaja - red in appearance, oily-slimy look, heaviness itching discharge blood stained-whitish in colour

Pittakaphaj - heavy, burning sensation, hot yellowish white discharge.

Vatapittaraktaj

Vatakapharaktaj

Kaphapittaraktaj

Vrana kruti - (shape of the ulcer) rectangluar, square, circuler and tringuler, shape of half moon and rarely different irregular shapes.

Vrana vastu - (tissues involved or base) skin, soft

tissues including muscles, blood vessels.......bones joints, viscus in the abdomen, vital point.

Vrana Gandha - (smell of the ulcer) smell that of ghee, oil, fat, pus, blood, acid, smell of copper mixed with curds or smell of dead body, foul smell.

Vran-Strav Discharge from ulcer in general - Serious watery, purulent, bloody, turmeric colourd, Reddish, yellowish red, brass coloured, blue colored, green, oily, dry, whitish.

Vataj Vrana - discharge is described as blackish, like dew, curds curds water, alkali water, meat wash or like pulak grass.

Pittaj ulcer - discharge like cow' urine, ash, decoction, oil, honey Shankha, gomedak mani.

Kaphaj Vrana - discharge like white butter, bonemarrow, groud sesame, coconut water, fat of the pig. It is cold, white slimy and more in quantity.

Tridoshas Vran - Coconut water, cucumber water, liver like, water baove kanji.

Vrana related to skin - water, serous little bad smell, related to.

muscle - ghee - coloured, white slimy and thick.

Siragat Vrana - if because of vessel cut - it is bloody if Nij vrana ripens - thin purulent, slimy, blackish and like dew, thready.

Realted to tendon - slimy, oily thick, realted to bone, Sanguinous, oily mixed with bone marrow.

Realted to joint - discharge appears on movement of the joint. It is slimy thready, sanguinous and frothy.

Koshthaget Vrana - ulcer related to abdominal viscus, discharge of blood, urine, faces, pus, water, bile depending upon viscus involved.

Vran Varna (Colour of the ulcer) Vataj Vran - ash, pigeon, bone like colour, blackish or black with abnormal colours.

Pittaj Vran - blue, green, blackish

Raktaja Vran - black, red or grey in colour

Kaphaj Vran - whitish, oily

Different - types of pains in vran, (ulcers), needleprick, brusting, beating, cutting, streching, like biting by ants, trembling, stiffness, heaviness, constriction, burning intense, heavey itching, loss of sensation, coldness etc.

SHUDDHA VRANA (Clean ulcer)

Floor of the ulcer looks like clean tongue, even surface, soft lusterful look, no discharge, no pains with red clean granulation tissue.

RUHYAMAN VRANA (Healing ulcer)

Edges of the ulcer show a pigeon color, without discharge and with beaded apperence. We find dry, thin, white growing skin layer on it.

ROODH VRANA (Healed ulcer)

Edges have come nearer. No depression and colour is like normal skin. No oedema or discharge.

Causes for non healing of the ulcer :

1. Degneration of muscle and tendan sheath
2. Worms
3. Fracture
4. Foreign body
5. Poison
6. Trauma white scratching
7. Uncessary bandaging
8. Excessive oily dressing

9. Indigestion
10. Excessive intake of food
11. Improper mixing of food materials.
12. Intake of food that does not suit.
13. Grief
14. Anger
15. Day time sleep
16. Exercise
17. Sex enjoyment
18. Trauma
19. Scraping of the ulcer
20. Lack of proper treatment
21. Lack of adequate sleep
22. Toxic gut (Gastro intestinal canal)
23. Intake of Alcohol
24. To take inadequate food
25. Fear

Complications of Vran

1. Cellulitis
2. Paralysis
3. Tetanus
4. Convulsions
5. Loss of consciousness
6. Severe pains
7. Fever, thirst lock jaw, cough, vomiting, diarrhoea, Hlicough, breathlessness

Ulcer heals easily and soon in persons with good digestive power and in young healthy individals. In small children and old patient it take long time for healing.

Ulcers related to anorectal region, perinium, forehead, neck, lips, back, ears, Scrotum, abdomen and area above clavicle heal easily.

Ulcer related to skin only heals easily, rounded, triangular and rectanglar ulcers heal easily.

Ulcer in eyes, near teeth, nose, ear, umbilicus, epigastric region, axilla, precordial region, breast and joints and ulcers throwing forthy, purulent, sanguinous discharge, with foreign bodies and difficult to heal.

Chapter : 6

Asthi-Bhagna (Fracture of the bone)

Formation of Asthi (ayurvedic view)

Asthi (Bone) consists of Pruthwi, Agni and Yayu-Mahabhutas. The previous dhatu viz med becomes dry to form Asthi. The cavity in the bone is filled up by oily meda viz Majja (Bone marrow) While describing the functions of bone viz holding different muscles and body tissues together sushrut has pointed out that though the skin and different other body tissues in the body become thin because of disease or starvation, the bony tissue does not reduce in size. Asthi nurishes the next dhau viz Majja.

Types of bones :-

1)	Kapal	-	Flat bones
2)	Ruchak	-	Teeth
3)	Tarun	-	Cartilages
4)	Walaya	-	Curved bones
5)	Nalak	-	Long cylindrical bones

Causes of fracture :- Fall from a height, severe pressure, different types of traumas.

Types of fracture :-

1) Sandhi-mukta Bhagna :- (Fracture with dislocation) In case of dislocation of a joint the muscles attached to the bones are stretched and pulled. During this process there is a small avulsion fracture of the bone at the attachment of the muscle and hence probably included in this fracture type.

2) Kand-Bhagna :- (Fracture of a long cylindrical bone)

Types of Sandhi-mukta Bhagna : -

i) Utpista :- There is a dislocation of articulating bones with fractures in them. There is swelling on either side, pain, There is upward displacement of dislocated bone.

ii) Vishlishta :- There is minimal dislocation. Swelling all around the joint but less. There is a severe pain all 24 hrs. in a day. There is formation of a hollow in between the bones.

iii) Vivartit :- Dislocating bones go away from each other. There is deformity and severe pain.

iv) Avakshipta :- The dislocation bone moves down. There are severe pains.

v) Atikshipta :- There is extreme dislocation of articulating bones with severe pain.

vi) Tiryak-Kshipta :- One of the articulating bones moves away. There is a severe pain.

vii) Kand-Bhagna :- (Clinical picture) Sweeling at the site of fracture, Tenderness (localised) deformity, painful movement of affected bone, Crepitus (as far as possible not to be elicited as it is severely painful) loss of movements. Patient is not comfortable in any position.

Type of Kand-Bhagna according to the deformity caused by fractured fragments.

i)	Karkatak	:-	Fractured fragments elevated giving a shape like a Crab.
ii)	Ashwakarna	:-	The broken parts of the fractured bone are much elevated and it looks like horse's ear.
iii)	Choornit	:-	Multiple small fragments at the site of fracture.
iv)	Pichchit	:-	Bone is compressed and hence becomes flat. There are cracks and lot of swelling.
v)	Asthichchhalit	:-	End of the bone, because of a fracture is just attached to the rest of the bone or totally gets separated from it.
vi)	Kand-Bhagna	:-	Complete fracture of a long cylindrical bone because of which the affected part becomes unstable.
vii)	Majjanugat	:-	One fractured fragment enters the central marrow cavity of the other, also called as impacted type.
viii)	Atipatit	:-	Complete fracture of the bone resulting into separation of the part from the body as in case of amputation.
ix)	Vakra	:-	There is no break but a bent in the bone. Greenstick fracture in children.
x)	Chhinna	:-	Partial fracture i.e. crack in one side of the cortex. The opposite

part of the cortex is intact.

xi) Patit :- Comminuted fracture more than two small or large fragments at the site of a fracture.

xii) Sphutit :- Multiple cracks in the bone but without flattening.

Prognosis :- Types 3, 7, 8, 10, 11 are described to be difficult to treat. Fractures in old, thin, weak, diseased patients and in children are difficult to treat. It is also difficult in patients suffering from lung tuberculosis, bronchial or cardiac Asthama, skin diseases & Compound or technically compound fractures. Osteoporotic bones, low appetite, constipation, retention of urine, fever are also responsible for difficult healing.

Comlications :- Delayed Union, Malunion, Non-union,

Treatment (In General) Parishek, Lep, Bandh.

Parishek :- It consists of slowly pouring of medicated decoction and oils hot or cold on the site of fracture considering the season and Dosha involved. This is used to lessen the pain. Herbs from Nyagrodhadigan, Laghupanchamool, Chakrataila are considered for this purpose.

Lep :- Application of a medicated paste on the site of a fracture. Powder of Red Sandal, Manjishtha, and Glyceriza Glabra, rice-flour are mixed together with 100 times washed Ghee and used for this purpose. This is used to reduce the swelling. The reduction of a fracture and application of a splint or plaster is only possible after the swelling is reduced. Lep is always of cool and cooling character which would bring under control the haemorrhage at the fracture site. The further procedure conssists of reduction of the fracture that is to bring the fragments in opposition. To give stability and rest to the fracture specific splints are used and they are called as Kusha.

After the allinment the site is to be wrapped in a cloth dipped in Ghee and then thin, broad sheets of the skin of certain trees like Kadamb, Peepal, Arjun, Umber, Vat, Palas etc. are used to give even support to the affected area to give immobilisation and rest to the fractured fragments. The bandaging should not be too tight or loose. In winter season this bandage is to be changed after every 7 days in summer after 3 days and in intermediate season after every 5 days. While changing this bandage the stability of the area is not to be disturbed.

Duration of immobilization :-

In children - one months

In young - two months

In old age - three months

Savran-Bhagna :- (Compound fracture)

All the care is taken to avoid infection and pus formation

Internal Medication :- Medicated Ghees, Babbultwak Choorna, Laksha-di Guggulu. Abha-di-Guggulu, Prawal-Bhasma, Calcipral of Ayurveda Rasashala are administered for better healing.

Abhyang (application of oil to body) Nasya (nasal medication) & Basti (Enema) using medicated oils is said to help the process of healing. Milk and wheat are very useful food items.

Chapter : 7

Agnikarma

(Cauterisation)

–Dr. G. S. Lavekar

"A therapy [Procedure] which is
carried by instruments made to hot,
or in which Agni is used as a measure
is called **Agni Karma**".

S.S. 12/1

Agni Karma is a non-operative therapy. It has got some relation with acupuncture therapy also.

As far as the application of therapcutic measures is concerned. It has been described that except for operative procedures the cauterination has got wide applicability in different discases.

Some times even after surgical operative procedures the cauteriation is necessary along with the surgical procedures.

In India the "Agnikarma Therapy' can be traced to the Atharviveda and Rigveda.

However, it is in Sushrut Sanhita we first come to across a systematic study of Agnikarma in view of applicability and methodology. Sushrut - Sanhita is the earliest treatise which deals with the Agnikarma in detail.

In Charak-Sanhita and vagbhata the Agni Karma is described in concise.

Sushruta deserves the credit of bringing the systematic study of the Agnikarma in surgical procedure.

No doubt that there is mention of Agnikarma in later books of Ayurveda such as Sharangdhara and Bhavaprakasha but they appear to be in very short and theoritical rather than practical.

Sushruta states that 'with regards to the surgical treatment actual cautery is said to be superior to Ksharn [Caustics] in as much as diseases heated with actual cautery do not reappear and because it can cure diseases which are incurable by medicines, instruments and caustics 5. 5. 12/3.

To this belief of the Sushruta may be compared to the following aphorism of the Hippocratos. "Those diseases which medicine do not care, the knief cures, those which iron cannot cure, fire cures and those fire cannot cure are to be reckoned wholly incurable." Syd. Vol. ii p. 774.

Agni Karma [thermal cautery] possesses some more advantages :

* As they do not give the idea of an operation, they shake the less the minds of the patients. So the patients are still less terrified by the application of cautery than by surgical measure.

* They are accepted with calmness with infinitely less efforts, than the action of the knife.

* Mortifying the tissues step by they give rise to no effusion of blood like inscision.

* Patients treated by Agnikarma do not require to remain in bed or to consider themeselves as patients.

Hospitolization is not that necessary in each and every case and more over early ambulation is easily advisable.

* Thee most important consideration of this therapy is that it affects less deeply the economy than the operation properly so called.

Dr. C.S. Lavekar
A. V. P. Ph. D. [Shalya Tantra]
[Poona University]
F I I M

(B)

Agnikarma Chikitsa

(Treatment by Theuraputic Burning)

In Sushruta Samhita (The old book of Indian Surgery) all Surgical and Parasurgical Tequnices are grouped in five groops.

(1) First is "**Shastra Karma**" that is operation by Sharp Instuments.

(2) Second is "**Agni Karma**" that means treatment by theuraputic burns.

(3) Thirdly there is "**Kshar Karma**" which is the treatment by application of Kshar.

(4) Forthly we have "**Bheshaja Karma**" there are herbal medicine to treat certain Surgical disorders.

(5) Fifth is "**Rakta Mokshan Karma**" Here by blood is taken out from the diseased park and Certain operations are avoied.

Thus Agnikarma, Ksharkarma, Bheshaj Karma, and Rakta-Mokshen Karma are para-Surgical tequniques.

Now we will see "**Agni Karma**" Chikitsa and its results in Short "**Agni Karma**"

(1) "**Purwa Karma**" (Pre-operative preperation). The Shalaka (Instument) made by five metals is kept on fire to get it red hot. The diseased part of the body is washed by "Triphala Kashay" (liquid) and the "Ghru Kumari swaras" is applied is the part.

(2) **Pradhan Karma (operation proper)** Make the

patient comfertable on the operation table in "Shalya karma Mandir" operation room, Five to twenty of "Samyak Dagdhas" (theuraputic Burn) are produced on diseased part to be trontod.

(3)"**Paschat Karma**" (Post operative Management) The "Dagdha Vrana" (Burn wounds) should be covered by Ghrut kumari Swaras" and "Bandhan" bandages should be applied.

By doing this treatment heat from shalaka (instrument) is transfered to the diseased part. This transfered heat increases the "**Dhatu Agni**" (Tissue Enzyme) which produces. "Pachan" (Digestion) of the "Dosha" (only kapha and Vata Dosha) which is the cause of disease.

The following diseases are trented by above tequnic and we got the results as noted below.

Diseases Treated	**Results in percents**
(1) Kadar (Corn)	70%
(2) Vranvastu mansutsed (keloid)	90%
(3) Granthi (Cyst)	60%
(4) Katishul and Katigrah (Sacralization & Lumbor Sponelings)	90%
(5) Pachurhul (Spin in Coleannum)	50%
(6) Chlocpeads (Heplamtheds) [only Kaphaj & Vataj]	70%
(7) Swetkushtha [leukodorma]	50%

(8) Vicharchika
[Eczema]
[only Kaphaj and Vataj] 70%

(9) Vranashotha
[Inflamation]
[In Amawastha &
Paohamanawatha] 90%

(10) Vatik Bahiarsha
[Thrombosed
Prolapsed Piles] 80%

Thus we are able to produce good and encoraging results by "Agni Karma Chikitsa" as shown above.

Dr. P.D. Gupta.
M.D. (Ay.)

(C)

Agnikarma (Cauterization)

The curable diseases which are not curved by drug, Kshar, surgery - could be cured by Agnikarma but incurable diseases could only be palliated for some time. Agnikarma was also used to stop bleeding during surgery and to excise the dead portion of the body.

Different materials which are used for this procedure are Pimpli (Piperlongum) – sheep-dung, cow's tooth, arrow, probe, are used in cases of diseases related to skin. Other suitable iron instruments are used in case of soft tissue.

Honey-Jaggery and fats (ghee, oil, tallow, marrow) are used at veins, muscles, bones and joints.

Diseaseses	Material used for Agnikarma
Moles warts, conjunctavitis	Pimpli, sheep-dung, cow's tooth,
Glaucoma, pain at-the site Of eyebrow, forehead and temple.	arrow, probe.
Cystic swelling tumour,	Needle, sharp probes prepared from
Pile, fistula, tubercular	Gold, silver, copper also - ghee,

lym-phadenitis, Elephantasis Hernia, Dacryocystitis, Dental sinus	Jaggery-Honey-wax, tallow

After discussions it is agreed that this cauterization is to be used to stop bleeding from soft-tissues, muscles, bones and joints and not to be used to irradicate totally the diseases at these places.

Agnikarma is not performed on Pitta-constitution personalities, when there is internal haemorrhage, perforations of gut, weak people and children, old patients, cowards and patients with multiple wounds.

Time for Agnikarma All seasons except Sharat and Greeshma, but in case of emergency in these seasons also.

Preparation of the patient. Patient is given slimy liquid light diet before. In case of urinary Calculus, haemorrhoids, fistula, Ascitis, diseases of mouth diet is not to be given before Agnikarma.

In case of ano-recal diseases patient is kept fasting for some time before the procedure.

There should be good light co-operative staff and good equipments.

Types of Agnikarma	Application
Circular	To excise tumour.
Bindu (Point)	To seal the bleeding point
Lines (on skin)	When more area is involved.
Flat application	When effect only limited to skin is Expected.
Halft moon or like	For muscles, joints

Signs of optimum - adequate **Dahankarma.** When skin is cauterised there is a specific noise like - Chur.r.r.r.r. there is a disagsreable smell colour of skin becomes gray, there is a little pain and swelling ulcer bcomes dry and contracted.

If adquate cauterization takes place at veinsand muscles - ulcer becomes black and elevated - bleeding stops.

When cauterization is performed at bone and joint - there occurs dryness, blackishness and stability at the site of wound above.

After adquate Dahankarma honey and ghee is freely applied to the injury which reduce pain and inflammation.

Accidental burns
(Itar-Dagdha)
(Pra-mad-Dagdha)

Because of dry or wet heat, boiling oils, strong corrosives, electricity, sun-rays.

Types

1) Plushta - Dagdha :- Superficial burn

Affected area becomes red first and then black. There is lot burning pain.

Treatment - Thin layer of a paste of powdered white sugar in little water applied on affected area will prevent blister formation.

White yolk of an egg mixed well with castor oil and if applied on affected area will reduce the pain and help early healing.

In this type it has been advised to avoid cooling application externally. External application should be warm in nature.

2) Durdagdha - Full thickness burns. There is blister formation. Lot of burning pain and redness which last for longer time. Possibility of pus formation inside the blisters.

External application of different creams, medicated ghee is indicated.

3) Samyag-dagdha - Not very deep burns. The colour of the skin looks like a ripe fruit

Treatment. External application of Vanshalochan, Plaksha, Sandle, Gairik and Guduchi along with ghee, in the paste form.

The paste of the flesh of different animals is also described. The other treatment as in Pittaj Vidradhi.

Ati-dagdha. Deep extensive burns involving muscles, blood vessels, bones and joints. Severe dehydration and hypovolemia, fever and unconsciousness. If at all patient recovers he gets contractures - chronic bonhealing ulcers.

Treatment. Dead soft tissue is excised. Pieces of rice are grounded and mixed with ghee to apply locally. The skin of Tindukti tree is powdered and along with the powder of pieces of earthern pot a paste is prepared for local application.

If patient survives after electrical burns, oliation in the form of Snehan, Abhyang and Parishek is pereformed.

In cases of suffocation by smoke, Vaman (Emesis) is advised. For that ghee, sugarcane juice, Grape juice, milk, sugar with water, are used. Patient is asked to gargle with sweet, salty, sour and pungent tasting decoctions. Nasal medication is also advised. Patient is given an easily digestible oily, non-irritating bland diet.

Modern surgery advices immediate replacement of fluids and electrolytes blood trasfusion,– Hypnotics and Medicines to prevent infection, care of the affected are, skin grafting and treatment of complications.

Chapter : 8

Yantras & Shastras (Surgical Instruments)

Yantra :- Any foreign body or damaged tissue or part of the body or thicknened secretions as in the form of calculi all known as shalyas. They are to be held (caught) with the help of some instruments and with or without the help of sharp instruments (shastrani) damaged structures are to be removed out of the body. These holding instruments are called as Yantrani.

These are also used to visnalise the disease process. There can be N number of Yantrani with more and more modifications. Six types of 101 such instruments are described.

Types :- Swastika Yantra (Atery forceps and similar instrument) about 18 Anguli in length with parts.

1) Mukha - (Tip & Catching portion)
2) Kantha - (Where two parts of the instrument are fixed)
3) Varang - (Grip area)

There are 24 types and they are named according to the appearance of their tips. The shapes of their tips look like the mouths of different birds and animals, out of which 9 are wild animals.

e.g. :- Lion, Tinger, bear, Leopard, Cat, Fox, Deer, Monkey, Crow, Owl, Heron, Stork, Falcon, Crane, Kite, etc.

Uses :- To catch hold of bleeding points.

To remove foreign bodies and calculi.

To drain the pus from abscess (Vidradhi)

To hold different tissues.

It is never to be applied to skin except in Circumcision.

2) Sandansha Yantra (Dissecting forceps, Thumb forceps)

Types :- 1) Sanigraha (with tooth at the tip)

2) Anigraha (without such tooth)

3) Vakradwibahu (with curved distal part)

Length :- First 2 types 16 Anguli

3rd types 6 X 2 Anguli

Uses :- To hold skin, muscle, vessels, nerves and many other soft parts in the body, while removing the parts and suturing the parts.

3) Tal Yantra : (Retractors)

One end or both the ends of the instrument are like fishmouth. This type of instruments are used to retract abdominal wall or deep cavities in the body during surgical procedures.

4) Nadiyantra

Hollow tubular instruments used for visualisation, suction, removal of foreign body, removal of secretions and discharges from the body like retained urine. Sushrut has described 20 sub types.

(1) Bhagandar Yantra Proctoscope

(2) Arshoyantra

(3) Vrana Yantra

(4) Basti Yantra - used to give enema

(5) Basti Netra

(6) Uttar basti Yantra - different types of catheters used to give enemas to be used in urinary bladder, uterus, vagina.

(7) Trochar and Canula

(8) Dhoom netra - used to inhale medicated smoke.

(9) Niruddha Prakasha Yantra - Urethral dilaters prepared from Iron, wood or Lac.

(10) Sannirudha-gud-Yantra-Anal dilator

(11) Alabu

(12) Ghati Yantra

(13) Shrunga (Horn of white cow) used for blood letting

(14) Kanthavalokanartha Nadi - instrument used to visualise throat.

(15) Anguli tranak - Thimble.

(16) Yoni - Vranekshan Yantra - Speculum to visualise vagina.

(17) Nadiswed - Netra - Tubular instrument used to administer steam.

Shalaka Yantra - there are different probes called as Shalaka Yantra to apply medicine, medicated thread, retraction of parts during surgery, for cauterization, dilatation, burring etc.

Hands of the surgeon are described to be the best instrument in shalyatantra, and following that the Kank - Mukha Swastik - Yantra.

Upa Yantrani (other objects) :- Not made up of the metal but could be used like surgical instruments as Rajju - (String), Venica, Patta - (belt), Valkal (Skin of the tree), Lata - (creeping plant) Vastra - (cloth), Mudger - Hammer, Flat of the hand & foot, digit, Tongue, Nail, Mouth, Hair, Kshara, Agni, medicine, magnet and processes like straining, spitting out, and Time, suppurative process, fear.

Sushrut has described 24 function to be performed by Yantras, mainly used for removal of foreign body Visualization, removal of discharges, diagnosis, correction, cleaning etc.

Yantra Gunas - (Good qualities of the instrument) Adequate - length, breadth, & thickness. Strong but with smooth mouth and tips. Good grip, and good shape.

Yantra Doshas - (Bad qualities) prepared from impure metal. Too large - long - or short, without good grip, loose, bent.

***

Shastra
(Sharp Instruments)

The instruments which can cut and cause more pain. As Shalyakarma (surgery) progressed, number of sharp instruments went on increasing in number.

According to Sushrut there were 20 sharp instruments.

(1)	Mandalagra	-	Long Khief like instrument with curved outside cutting sharp edge. Used for cutting & scraping.
(2)	Karapatra	-	Saw used to cut the bone.
(3)	Vrudhipatra	-	Surgical khief with sharp blade used for incision, excision.
(4)	Nakha Shastra	-	To remove nails, to take incisions, to puncture, for scraping.
(5)	Mudrika	-	Sharp short instrument to be worn on index finger, used to take incisions in the mouth and throat.
(6)	Utpalpatrak	-	Sharp end of this instrument is like the petal of a Lotus flower, used for incision and excision and Siravyadh.
(7)	Ardha-dhar	-	Half the length of this khief is sharp.
(8)	Soochi	-	Different types of suturing needles with round body or

			cutting body used to suture different tissues in the body. Eyeless needles were also sued.
(9)	Kushapatra	-	Sharp pointed knief with double edge used for blood letting procedure. Also was described to be used to incise abscesses in an Elephant.
(10)	Atimukh	-	Tip of the instrument is like the mouth of Crane. Used for blood Letting.
(11)	Shararimukh	-	Pair of scissors.
(12)	Antarmukh	-	Used for blood letting.
(13)	Trikoorchak	-	Used for blood letting.
(14)	Kutharika	-	(Chisel) used to chisel out the bone.
(15)	Vreehimukh	-	(Trochar) used for Siravyadh Vidradhi-bhedan, Paracentesis.
(16)	Ara	-	For Vidradhi-bhedan (To puncture abscess cavity)
(17)	Vetas-Patra	-	Siravyadh
(18)	Badish	-	Just like mandalagra but with inside cutting sharp edge.
(19)	Danta-shanku	-	Dental instrument to clean the teeth.
(20)	Eshani	-	A long probe with one sharp pointed end. Used for probing and Bhedan.

Average length of shastra is 6 Angule.

Instrument must possess a good sharp edge.

Payana :– After the manufacturing of a sharp

instrument when it is red hot it is to be dipped in Alkali, water and oil to make it more sharp. This process is called Payana. The small children and coward patients fear the sight of sharp instrument. In these patients some other objects like Glass, Leech, Fire, Kshar (Alkali) different rough leaves, hair, fingers, some special stones, skin of bamboo are used. They are called **Anushastrani.**

[Reference : Ayurveda workshop 1998]

Chapter 9

Surgical Ethics And Ayurved

Dr. S. I. Nagral

Surgery then known as Shalyatantra in Ashtanga Ayurved, was considered the first and the foremost amongst the prevent specialities. Sushrut, the Father of Surgery, was undoubtedly a great surgeon. After going through the works of Sushrut, one comes to the conclusion that the Art and Science of surgery had advanced to unimaginable heights. The ethical principles enunciated and practised were of the highest order. Unfortunately, because of unforeseen circumstances, it lagged behind and the continuity of the tradition get interrupted.

The word Ethics literally means – The science of moral values. Medical ethics refers to the code i.e., guiding principles and accepted rules of behaviour for the medical men with the patients, Government and among themselves. Here in this talk, I am using the word - Surgical Ethics with reference to the ideal ways of behavior in relation is Teaching, Training, Professional services, Quackery etc. as prescribed by celebrated authorities like Sushrut, Charak, Vagbnat and Kashyap.

Ayurved, the science of Life, has a rich tradition and is found to be of great relevance even today. In words of Maharshi Charak – "There is no end to the learning of Ayurved. Hence you should cautiously and constantly devote yourself to it. In addition, you should increase your professional skill by learning from others without being jealous. The intelligent would regard the whole world as their teacher, wheras the unintelligent would think the same as their enemy."

He stressed the importance of practical and discriptive knowledge of anatomy, physiology and pathology as a basis for learning surgery.

The authority to practice surgery was specifically assigned to only those who were experienced in the art and science of surgical and para-surgical procedures.

No one was allowed to start practice unless he has undergone the rsegular course of studied, seen and performed the operations himself, succeeded in the appropriate test and obtained the permission of the governing authority. He was expected to have proper apparrel and observe the rules of clealiness like clipping of nails and hair. Based of the philosophy of treating the patients only on humanitarian ground without desiring financial or personal gains and considering gift of life as supreme gift, balanced mind wishing good to everyone without trying to showoff and accompanied by able assistants. Practical residential training was mandatory in addition to the regular course of studies.

Generally a surgeon was expected to keep abreast of knowledge, take part in scientific debates and discussions, observe the allied sciences and take training from the concerned specialist. "Boldness, swiftness, sharpness of instruments, no sweating or trembling of hands and decisiveness, are the praiseworthy qualities of a surgeon at the time of operation" are mentioned as special qualities.

"Always pray for the wellbeing of all creatures. Fullest efforts should be tried to cure the sick throughout day and night, however, you may be engaged. Have no ill-feelings towards a patient even for the sake of your living or life. You should not commit adultery even in thought, nor convert other's possessions. Try to be simple and modest in your dress as well as in appearance. Don't be a drunked. Neither do a sin a nor associate yourself with a sinner. Your language should be gentle, pure, righteous, courteous, worthy, true, wheresome and moderate. You should take your past experience the account. Always try to increase your knowledge and equipment. Don't boast too much of your knowledge, even though you may possess it. Others get offended by the boastfulness of even capable persons" preached Maharshi Chatak as requisites of an ideal doctor.

Similar ideals regarding equipment, nursing staff attendans, drug etc. were specified.

Maharshi Sushrut while implementing the programme of training emphasized on adequate theoritical and practical learning. In his own words........."He who knows theory only, but is not proficient in practical work, gets..........bewildered on being confronted with a patient in the same way as a coward feels on the battle field. On the other hand, he, who is good, in practical work because of his boldness, but lacks theoritical knowledge, is not respected in the cultured society; actually he deserves punishment by the government. Both these types of persons can not be considered as experts and they are not capable of doing their work properly; they posses onesided knowledge only can be likened to birds who have one wing only. Only that intelligent person who knows both theory and practical work is capable of obtaining success in the same way as only two wheeled chariot move majestically on the battle-field."

Special mention regarding the behaviour towards

ladies is made by Maharshi Kashyap as - "he should not cut jokes with ladies or even with female servants; he should not call them by such names which appear mix up and be friendly with them. No offering of any kind should be accepted from a woman without the knowledge of her husband or guardian; he should not enter the place without previous information."

While describing the detail of management of surgical cases, detailed description regarding the preparation of patients like history taking, physical examination, proper diagnosis, assessment general condition, was stressed. In fact, specific mention is made regarding the abnormalities in the body likely to adversely affect the operative procedures team for conducting the operation safely and smoothly, is given lot of importance. Details regarding the operative procedures are described by incorporating the correct choice of operation, type of incision, the necessity of replacement of fluid, adequate and proper haemostais and the final check up before closing the wound.

Since the concept of transmission of infection was known to Maharshi Sushrut, he had strictly implemented the aseptic and antiseptic measures. The warning signs of impending shock were stressed and fluid replacement was advocated. While stressing the importance of blood replacement and arrest of bleeding the mention is made as – "Blood is the origin of body; the body totally depends upon it, hence every attempt must be made to preserve it. In other words, blood is equivalent to life itself. Pure blood imparts strength, complexion and a healthy life to the individual. Actually the whole mode of a person depends upon blood." The surgeon was expected to maintain high proficiency in the post-operative management by taking care of the patient particularly that of the wound.

Maharshi Sushrut has professed regarding the experimental surgery too. He has condemned the quacks and quackery in clear terms....'The practitioner who does not know medical procedures and surgical techniques is Quack. Such a person kills the people due to his greediness, and survives only because of the negligence of the governing authority. Surgery by him who opens an unripe swelling, as also of his who neglects the ripe abscess is based on indecision and both of them should be regarded as Quacks. Medicines equivalent even to nector when prescribed by quacks, may act like fatal weapons, lightening or poisons; hence one should avoid Quacks."

Special mention is made regarding the ethical behavior towards the terminally ill and emergency patients.

In the monumental volumes of Samhitas of Ayurved, Surgical Ethics is refered at many places and very many times. All that one needs to do is to imbibe and incorporate the spirit and the contents into the requites of Surgical Training and Practice today.

Ref. Sushrut Samhita

Surgical Ethics in Ayurveda by Dr. G. D. Singhal and Pt. D. S. Gaur.

[Reference : MUSING AYURVEDA 1992]

Chapter : 10

Philosophical, practical & Pragmatic approach of Sushrut for Holistic health care

Dr. S. I. Nagral

Sushrut is a pioneer surgeon and a legend in the world of surgery. He was a leading figure in the renowne dinstitution headed by Divodas Dhanvantari and acquired tremendous amount of knowledge and experience along with this esteemed colleagues namely Aurabhra, Aupadhenava, Karvaveerya, Gopurakshita, Nimi etc. As a leader of Dhanvantari sampraday, he preached and practised the art and science of surgery and documented the medical science prevelent then in an excellent manner. It is available today as Sushrut Samhita serving the generation of surgeons as a treasure of guidelines narrated in the form of precise stanzas arranged in different sections spread over 120 chapters. Even after hundreds of years of publication, the memorable volume is serving the medical profession as the relevent rellable and resourceful document useful in day to day practice and teaching.

Let me share with you a, few of his thoughts particularly the ones related to Holistic Health Care.

One is considered to be healthy. If the vital components of the body namely Doshas (Neuroumous), Agni (Digestion capacity), Dhatus (Tissues) and malas (Excretary substances) are regulated and are in equillibrium along with the related soul, armonious organs and cheerful mind..........said sushrut.

Maintainance of health in the healthy and curring the disease in the afflicted are mentioned as main aims of Ayurveda i.e. Science of life. I consider that each fundamental thoughts will contribute significantly to holistic health care.

It is a wellknown fact that the physician, Drugs, Nursing faculty, and Patients form four main pillars of health care system. If each one of them possess ideal qualities, the system will bear success. In the actual management of patient, the science is like a lighthouse which illuminates the environment, but the physician has to use his own vision in each and every case supplemented by drugs and nursing staff.

The most important among the four is the physician who is the guilding force. Naturally the would by physician has to be selected properly trained well, guideda by broad principles and supplemented by experiences, proper personnel, drugs and amenities.

In selecting the candidates, care was taken to see that he comes from cultured family, is of proper age, possess good moral character, courage, politeness, enthusiasm, sharp memory, adequate intelligence and knowledge coupled with good personality and physical fitness. Special mention is made to see that he does not possess any of adverse qualities.

The teacher is supposed to be capable to guide, disciplined possessing physical and mental ability with vast experience in the field and is willing to undertake the task.

Sushrut was mainly a surgeon, but an excellent teacher basically preparing the general physicians and the specialists as surgeons. He was a committed, capable and conscious individual, but precise, practical and firm in decisions.

While mentioning many qualities which a surgeon should possess, he said 'boldness, swiftness, sharpness of instruments, no sweating and trembling of hands and confidence are the essential qualities of a surgeon (Particularly while operating). [2]

Further one he mentions............

Practice can be started only after having read and thoroughly studied the science of medicine, having winessed the operative procedures and performed the same under the supervision, having passed the appropriate examination and after obtaining registration from the competent governing authorities.

The practitioners should keep short hairs, clipped nails. Personal hygience and cleanliness should have been taken care of. He should wear white and sober dress.

On his visits, he should move about with a cool and balanced mind, wishing everybody good, without trying show off and with an attitude to help all and should be accompanied by an able assistant.

Basically he should keep in mind that a person who studies one type of science only can not arrive at proper conclusions, hence a physician should try to learn as many relates sciences as possible.[3] In order to be able to understand the related sciences whose reference has to be taken in medical science because of necessity, one should listen to the lectures given by the specialists of that branch as it is not possible to include all branches of science in one subject.

With a view to keep continuity with the proper of quiring knowledge and broaden the outlook, one should keep on studying the subject regularly, take part in scientific discussions, observe the allied sciences and take training form the specialists of those branches.[4]

While talking of training Sushrut emphatically mentioned that..........

He who knows theory only but not good in practical work, gets bewildered on being confronted with a patient in the same way as a coward feels on the battle field.[5]

On the other hand, he who is good in practical work because of boldness, but lacks in theoritcal knowledge, is never respected in the civilised society, in fact he deserves to be punished by the governing authorities.[6]

Both these type of persons can not be considered as experts and are not capable of carrying on their work properly; they possess one sided knowledge only and be likened to a bird who has one wing only.[7]

Only that intellegent person who masters both theory and practical work is capable of obtaining success in the same way as a two sound wheeled chariot moves majestically on the battle field.[8]

Talking about the relations with the patients he stressed that the patient may doubt his relatives, his sons and even parents, but has full faith in the physician. He gives himself up in the physician's hands and has no misgivings about him. Therefore the physician becomes dutybound to look after him as his own sons.

In the vary similar ways, the practitioner is advised to deal with the society, patient's relatives, colleagues, governing authorities etc. in a dignified and ethical manner. Such preaching is bound to motivate a practitioner to behave in a philosophical way which in turn certainly helps to approach the health care system in holistic manner.

Before undertaking the actual treatment, the physician

is adviced to established rapport and win confidence of the patient and is expected to note the following particulars specially by interrogating him namely.....residence, climate of the locality, community, articles which suit his constitution and those of which he is sensitive, onset and history of present illness. In addition to normal enquiry, the intensity and nature of pain, general health, appetite, digestions, bowel movements, micturition and the duration of illness etc. are to be noted.

All forms of treatments should be undertaken only after full consideration of the Intensity of the discase, the general condition of the patient and the digestive & metabolic powers.

Lot of importance was given to the power of resistance. For example wound are known to heal normally in young, strong, and in patients with good resistance and mental ability. It is really a pleasure to treat a patient who possesses such qualities.

Unless taken care of a patient with poor general condition, goes from bad to worse and later on he may go beyond possibility of recovery. As life depends on power of resistance, every effort should be made to protect it and increase it.

When death appears to be certain by conservative treatment and surgery offers the doubtful hope, it should be carried out after taking the consent of the guardians in order to justify himself. Elaborate preparation of the patient was undertaken to facilitate the operative procedure, to smoother the recovery and to prevent complications.

Effects of injury and infections resulting in applications were taken into consideration while implementing the operative procedure by sterilising the instruments properly, handling the tissues by proper dissection, reconstruction and alignment.

Importance of replacement of fluids and blood tranfusion were noted and they were undertaken routinely.

Special methods were employed for proper haemostasis. Post operative check up was a must before closing the cavity. It was stressed that dust hairs, nails, loose bones and such other foreign material when found in the wound, should be removed. It they are not removed they will produce different types of pains and extensive suppuration. Care of the wound was undertaken for maintainance of function and acsthetic appearance.

Apart from the routine academic training, the candidate was expected to undergo the practical surgical training called Yoga kriya. Sushrut said 'Even if one is wellversed in all aspects of science, the disciple should necessarily undergo the process of Yoga.' He should be trained invarious lines of treatment like location, excision etc, because the learned even, not trained in practicals prove incapable in undertaking surgery.

The process of training is well designed and appropriate exercises are carried out on various substances including the tissues of the dead animals to make him conversent with the basic surgical procedures like Astha Vidha Shastrakarmas (eight types of basic surgical procedures.) To make the candidate proficient in the art and science of surgery, was the main consideration in the programme of Yogya.

Postoperatively it is expected that the patient should be rest in a comfortable bed attended by well trained nursing staff, sympathetic & affectionate friends and relatives who should be good conversationists too. Apart from the care of the wound locally and creating healthy & cordial atmosphere, special emphasis was suggested on maintainance of vitality. Based upon the season and the constitution, the drugs and the diet were planned. Cordial atmosphere, proper care of the wound, symptomatic management, care of putrition and vitality, monitering and management of cos pications, early mobilisation, social rehabilitation etc, were the main consideration, in the post operative management. It was not just the drug therapy helping the patient to recover, mainly it is the physical, mental, social and psychological care to hasten the process of the recovery.

Being pragmatic in approach Maharshi Sushrut condemned quackery in clear terms. He narrates.....

The physician who learns the science of medicine under the guidance of recognised teacher and regularly takes the practical training and thou practiscs medicine is the real physician; other are quacks.[9]

The practitioner who does not know the medical procedures (massage, heat therapy, medications, stomach wash by vomiting techniques and enema etc.) and surgical techniques (incision, excision, tapping, currettage, sounding, probing etc.) is a quack. Such persons kill the people because of greediness and survivies only because of the negligence of governing authorities.

He who knows when the abscess is unripe, has a tendancy towards ripening or is fully ripe is the doctor. Others are quacks. Surgery by him who opens an unripe swelling, also of his who neglects a ripe abscess, is based on indecision and both of them should be regarded as quacks.

Medicines even equivalent to nector when prescribed by quacks may act like fatal weapons, lightening or poisons. Hence one should always avoid quacks.[10]

Some of the methods of treatment like Ksharasutra, Ksharakarma, Jalokavacharan etc are proving to be highly effective and quite simple to implement. Not only that they are useful in cases where surgery is contraindicated because of the presence of dreaded disease or low general condition but they are observed to be effective in all routine cases. In fact some of these methods are proving very popular, cost effective, simple and are associated with least complications.

In emergency cases, the doctor is advised not to apply the routine methods of treatment, instand he should act as if his own house is on fire.

As I said earlier, Sushrut Samhita is treasure of knowledge and experience narrated in a lucid manner and acceptable to many in the field from junior medical students to senior practitioners and mature teaching faculty. The essence of knowledge of medical science is prescribed in a precise and pragmatic manner. The more you rad it, you feel like reading again. It always appears fresh and latest in concepts.

Precisely we say that harmonious existance of physical, physiological, psychological and spiritual entity is healthy. This state does get disturbed by environmental, social and personal factors. In actual lifesigns of good health are observed by nothing normal and physical and mental growth, healthy complexion, virtous behaviour, satisfied expression, cordial interpersonal relations, not being in race for power, paisa and publicity and not a victim of anger, ego, greed, temptation, prejudice etc.

The relief of miseries of disease of disease are observed as of happiness. Change in voice complexion, body figure and strength, regaining normal taste, desire to eat, proper digestion and assimilation, undisturbed sleep, proper expulsion of flatus, urine faces, cheerful mind, sharp memory.

To achieve the healthy status and to treat the diseases, Maharshi Sushrut has adopted excellent methods of training programme of health personnel, implementation of regimens, quality drugs, proper diet, social behaviour etc. By implementing the multifaceted programme, he has proved beyond doubt that holistic approach to health is the right way.

References :

१. समदोषः समाग्निध समधातुमलक्रियः।
प्रसन्नात्मेन्द्रियमनाः इतस्थ इत्यभिधीयतो।।

२. शोर्यमाशुक्रिया शस्त्रतैक्ष्ण्यम् अस्वेदवेपथू।
असम्मोहश्च वैद्यस्य शस्त्रकर्माणि शस्यते।।

३. एकं शास्त्रमधीयानो न विद्यात् शास्त्रविश्चयम्।
तस्माद् बहुश्रुतः शास्त्रं विजानीयात चिकित्सकः।।

४. सतताध्ययनं वादः परतन्त्रातलोनम्।
तद्विद-आचार्य सेवा च बुद्धिमेधाकरो गणः।।

५. यस्तु केवल शास्त्रज्ञः कर्मस्वपरिनिष्ठितः।
स मुह्यत्यातुरं प्राप्य प्राप्य भीरुरियाहवम्।।

६. यस्तु कर्मसु निष्णातो धाष्टर्यात् शास्त्रबहिष्कृतः।
स सत्सु पूजां नाप्नोति वद्यं चार्हति राजतः।।

७. उभौ एतौ स्वकर्मणि अनिपुणौ असमर्थौ ।
अर्धवेदधरौ एतौ एकपक्षाविव द्विजौ।।

८. यस्तूभयज्ञो मतिमान् स समर्थोऽर्थसाधने।
अहित कर्म निर्वोढुं द्विचक्रः स्यन्दनो यथा।।

९. शास्त्र गुरुमुखोद्‌गीर्णं आदायोपास्य चासकृत्।
यः कर्मः कुरुते वैद्यः रा वैद्योऽन्ये तु तस्कयः।।

१०. औषध्योऽमृतकल्पास्तु शस्त्राशर्विवषोपमाः।
भयन्त्यज्ञैः उपहृता तस्माद् एताव विवर्जयेत्।।

Chapter : 11

Immortal Ayurvedic Surgical Principles And treatment

Prof. : R. B. Gogte,

Charak, Sushruta & Wagabhata are the god fathers of Ayurved, period near about 2000, 1500 & 500 years B.C., have associted the surgical principles and treatment which is in consistance with Modern Surgical Principles and treatment. Sushruta has done nice detailing about it.

In this short speech I will give you few examples.

1) Suturing of a traumatic wound

Ayurved states that all traumatic incised wounds, surgical incisions to cure the disease should be sutured immediately. Suturing helps quick healing. It reduces time of hospitalisation also. (Ref. V. S. 29. 49. 46 & S. C. 1. 45)

If for some reasons suturing is not possible, bring the edges together and give a bandage. (Ref. C. c. 25/ 65)

2) Contraindications for Suturing the Wound

Active bleeding inside the wound, suspected foreign body in the wound, wound contained with dirt, acids, alkalies, poisons etc. or a wound through which the air is expelling like in respiratory tract injuries, you should not suture the wound. (Ref. S. S. 25/16.26 & V.S. 29/ 49.53)

If you want to suture the wound, stop the bleeding, remove the foreign body and suture.

Suturing Material

Cotton, Thread, Jute or Tag thread, Muscle fascial strips, ext. skin of the trees, tendrils of the trees were used. The use of hairs is also described esp. for the wounds on the face. The tongs of the black Ants's are also been described for the wounds on gastrointestinal tract.

Except Muscle fascial strips other material is non absorbable. It is just like the catgut which we use in Modern Surgery. Tong of the black Ants is just like Mickel's clips. (Ref. S. s. 25/16 and A. s. U. 17/47)

Needles

Four types of needles are described. The Modern name of it is given infront of it.

Aayata	Vritta.	Straight	round body
Aayata	Tryasra	Straight	cutting
Dhanur	Vakra	Curved	
Nigoodha	Pasha.	Eyeless / Atramatic	

Dhanur Vakra (curved) needle is to be used for deeper structures

(Ref. A. S. S. 34, S. S. 25/23, 26 & S. S. 25/23-26)

Types of Suturing

Four types are been described. The modern name is given infront of it.

Vrijugranthi	Simple Stitch
Gophanika	Matress

Anuvelitaka Spiral
Tunnasevani Subcutuicular
(*Ref. S. S. 16. 28*)

How to suture the Wound

Stiching should not be done too near to the wound edge nor too away from the edge of the wound, as they produce over hanging of the skin edge and pain resp.

In modern medicine 1 c.m. distance from the edge of the wound and one c.m. distance between the two sutures is ideal, only, in case of Vrijugranthi. (Simple Stich)

Secondary Suturing

All old non infected incised wounds should be resutured again as it cut shorts the healing process. This should be done only after scraping the wound eage till it bleeds freely.

Same principles are followed in modern surgery. (Ref. V. S. 29. 49. 56)

Sutures to be removed on Seventh day.

Sutures are to be removed after seven days as all non infected wounds must heal in seven days. It is consistant with Dhattpatti. Dnyaya, in Ayurved. In modern surgery sutures, are removed in between 5th to 10th day generally on 7th day. (Ref. A.S.U. 31)

Methods of Controlling the bleeding.

Ayurved gives importance for controlling the bleeding as blood or Rakata is (Jeevan) life giving to the patient. Four methods are described to control the bleeding which are the same in modern medicine also.

i) Sandhan - By astringents, By Styptics, By ligation of bleeding points and by tight bandage / Tourniquet. (Ref.

V. S. 27. 43. 44)

ii) Skandan - Cold application, refrigeration or internal sheet medicines.

This is achieved by putting cold water sponges on the wound, application of Algae, ice etc. or sheeta lepas, putting the patient in cool place. (Ref. s. s. 14. 36)

iii) Pachan - Removal of a clot of blood or slough.

This method is used for bleeding in infected wound where the slough prevents the contraction of blood vessel or where the clot in the mouth of vessel prevents contraction of the blood vessel. This was done by Ksharas. Now a days the Ksharas been replaced by hydrogenperoxide. (Ref. s. s. 14. 36)

iv) Dahan - by heat Cautury.

The bleeding is stopped by touching the bleeder by red hot shalaka. In modern surgery Electrically operated coagulation cautary is used for the same purpose. Ayurved advocates this method to be utitlised as last report. (Ref. s. s. 36. 43)

Concept of bleeding and coagulation time

This concept has been described in Ayurveda in the Chapter of plastic surgery, the Chinna Chikitsa. If there is defective mechanism as askandi (prolonged clotting time) as we get in Vata, Pitta doosta Rakata and Chirasravi (prolonged bleeding time) as we get in Kaphadooshata Rakata, no plastic surgery is to be done as it prevents primary healing. (Ref. S. S. 14.21)

Peritoneal lavage in peritonitis / contaminated peritoneal cavity (Chidrodar Chikitsa)

Due to bull horn injury, Stab wounds on the abdomen or due to perforation of an ulcer, appendix or M. Diverticulum there is soiling of the peritoneal cavity due to infected material like dust, dirt, gastro intestinal secretions or bacterias-Ayurved states that after suturing, the injury of the gastro-intestinal tract, the peritoneal cavity should be well washed to remove and type of foreign or infected material. This washing was done with milk.

In Modern Surgery the same i done by using Liquid Metrogyl Saline or Distilled Water. (Ref. S. C. 14/17)

Wounds having a tendency to heal late.

Patients having Madhumeha (Diabetes), Mahakushtha (Leprosy), Shosha (Tuberculosis) or sounds contaminated with poinsons have a tendency to heal late. (Ref. S. S. 23)

Concept of Hypoprotenaemia & Wound healing

According to Ayurveda wound healing depends upon the Mansa Dhatu (Muscle Proteins) which is uplepaka. If the mansadhatu i.e., proteins are defecient, eventhough the wound is clean, non infected the wound refuses to heal. In this Particular condition a diet containing high protein is indicated. This Karma is described as Udasadan. This condition is similar to non healing of a wound due to hypoproteinaemia in modern Surgery.

Ayurveda advocates chicken or mutton rich diet.

(Ref. S. C. 81. 83 and C. C. 25. 50)

Cysts to be removed with their capsule.

All the encapsulated cysts or tumours should be removed with capsule, otherwise recurrence is possible. (Ref. C. C. 12. 82. 83)

Excision of omentum (Medovarti)

In modern surgery the omentum if to be excised, is ligated first and then excised as the vessels are unsupported and are likely to bleed.

In Ayurveda they have described the same. Transfix the omentum and excise it with red hot knife. Red hot knife prevents bleeding and infection which is another advantage in Ayurveda. (Ref. S. C. 2. 45 & I. A. S. 3.31/234)

Fallen tooth to refix immediately and Feed the patient with Kamal Nal - Loutus stem - straw

Sometimes in accident or due to direct blow on teeth they fall out with the root. Ayurved states that such teeth or tooth should be immediately replaced in the socket, biting to be stopped and Fedding should be done, by stem of lotus (like straw) for 7 to 10 days.

Replacement should not be done in old people or the tooth which was loose before trauma. (Ref. S. c. 3.41.43)

Abscess to be incised adequately and counter incisions to be taken if necessary.

Abscess should be incised adequately. The incision should be straight and big enough so as not to leave any collection of pus in the abscess cavity.

If one incision is not sufficient take as many incisions as necessary so that no pus is left behind. These are counter incisions according to modern surgery. (Ref. S. S. 5/9 & S. S. 5/11.12)

These are the few illustrative examples and so many other could be illustrated. They are still practiced. I am very much thankful to you, Dr. P. H. Kulkarni and organisation of this programme to give me this nice opportunity.

[Reference : MUSING AYURVEDA 1992]
[International Conference on Ayurveda]

Chapter : 12

Scope and Role of Ayurved in Modern Anaesthesia

Dr. D. P. Puranik

No discovery ever made in Medicine has proved more beneficial to the human race than the discovery of Anaesthesia, not only because it has alleviated the fearful path of surgery but also because the whole structure of Modern Medicine has drawn strength from its success, and surgery has been able to accomplish, with its aid, a greater advance in the last century than in all the preceding millenia.

Status of Anaesthesia in Ayurved -

If we look back, it is seen that in ancient time, in India, the medical branches other than anaesthesia were much developed and advanced. Ayurvedic books and literature reveal full and detail knowledge about shalya-shalakya tantra (Surgery, E.N.T., Ophthalmology), Chikitsa (Medicine) narrate the different methods of operations in detail. Unfortunately very little knowledge and few references are available about the methods in Sammohan Shastra. (Anesthesiology). The probable reason for this unavailability seems to be that the repeated aggressions on India might have destroyed the concerned Grantha or might have stolen these Grantha.

No specific drugs are described in 'Ayurvedic books' which were used as Anaesthetic drugs at the time. Still some references as to how anaesthesia was conducted at that time are available.

Giving of *'Madya' (Alcohal)* in large doses to the patient undergoing surgery so as to achieve a stage of *"Vish-Madyaj Murchha"* was a very popular method. (Ref. Sushrut) 'Matta Shastram Na Badhate'.

Use of specific powder, called as *"Mohachurna"* was also known (Ref. - Use of 'Mohachurna' by Ashwini Kumar - Bhojprabandh). This resembles inhalation type of anaesthetic from modern anaesthesia.

Use of *Madhur* and *Snigdha Ahar* for the patients who are not accustomed to alcohol to increase their tolerance towards pain was one of the methods.

Snehan and Swedan Vidhi - prior to surgery to achieve a stage of muscular relaxation was also customary.

Use of *'Nidrajanan and Vedanasthapan'* (Sedatives and Analgesic) dravya, prior to surgery was also a popular method to quieten the patient undergoing surgery.

Present Status of Modern Anaesthesia -

Modern anaesthesia in recent times, especially, after two world wars, advanced very fast and so, scope of surgery has been much extended due to it. The modern anaesthesia, has not only kept pace with rapid advances made in surgery but has in many instances enabled these advanced to be made.

Anaesthesia is now much safer and more pleasant for the patient than it was 50 years ago. Factors contributing to the improvement include fuller understanding of physiology and pharmacology, better pre-operative assessment and preparation of patients, introduction of patent drugs like Fentanye, Pentazocine, Morphine derivatives for preanaesthetic medication, use of potent anaesthetic like Fluothane, and anaesthetic gas–nitrous oxide, etc.

All these have made the anaesthesia very palatable. Introduction of regional analgesia without affecting patients consciousness, new intravenous anaesthetic agents, muscle relaxants, art of resuscitation, Mechanical ventitators, monitoring equipments and perfection in blood gas analysis, all these factors have changed anaesthesia into a discipline.

Scope and Role of Ayurved in Modern Anaesthesia :

Now the question arises whether Ayurved has any place in modern anaesthesia? Can Ayurved contribute in its own right in present status of anaesthesia? If answer is 'yes', in what way?

Though Modern anaesthetists have greatly imporved the quality of their work, morbidity and mortality associated with anaesthesia are far from satisfactory. Pre-anaesthetic anxiety and apprehension, post-operative complications and sequel stills persist undersired side effects of these drugs is also a problem to be solved.

Opportunities for research in Anaesthesiology are boundless. After all, the mechanisms by which general anaesthetics act are still unknown nearly 150 years after their first use.

So the stalwarts and young inspiring research scholars in the field of Ayurved determined to assess and prove the utility of certain Indigenous drugs having anaesthetic properties) for the aid of Modern anaesthesia.

Clinical and Laboratory trials were given to Ayurvedic drugs possessing anaesthetic properties to evaluate their utility at pre-anaesthetic stage, during anaesthesia and post anaesthetic recovery stage.

All these research studies were carried out at different institutes and with collaboration of and under supervision of modern aneshetists. At may instances same drugs were given trials at different Institutes adopting different methodology.

The study results were very promising and encouraging in most of the projects undertaken and in some instances Ayurvedic drugs proved to be more satisfactory and useful than the established modern drugs.

In support of all the previous statements and comments, this will be a right occasion to have brief review regarding research work and projects carried out at different Ayurvedic Institutes in India regarding the subject.

i) Study of Role of 'Parasik Yawani' as pre-anaesthetic tranquillizer (Hyocymus-reticulata).

Work was carried out for Fellowship in Anaesthesia at Pune (Tilak Ayurved Mahavidyalaya) in 1978.

(same drug was given trial at B.H.U.)

ii) Study of "Suvarna-sootshekar" as antiemetic for post anaesthetic vomitting (1971).

Study was carried out for F.F.A.M. at Pune. (Tilak Ayurved Mahavidyalaya).

iii) Study of 'Nidroday Rasa' as pre-anaesthetic hypnotic.

Study was carried out at (Tilak Ayurved Mahavidyalaya, Pune) for F.F.A.M. (1982).

iv) Changes in C.V.S. in relation to Prakruti during General Anaesthesia (1978).

v) Anaesthesia and study of certain Indigenous drugs credited for anesthetic properties - M.D. (Ayu.), G.A.U., Jamnagar (1980).

vi) Studies on certain Indigenous Drugs as Anaesthetic Agents.

vii) Pre-anaesthetic Medication in Indigenous drugs for Local Anaesthesia.

(M.D.) (Ayu.), B.H.U. (1983)

viii) A clinical study of Sharpunkha with additional study of its anaesthetic action.

M.S.A.M. (G.A.U.), Jamanagar (1971)

x) Free Fatty Acid and Blood Glucose studied after the use of Jalanimba and Shankapuship as pre-anaesthetic agents.

(M.D. (Ayu.) B.H.U., Varanasi (1978).

xi) Study of Ayurvedic Medicine for post spinal headache.

F.F.A.M., Potdar Hospital, Bombay - 1980.

All these research studies definitely indicate the involvement and usefullness of Ayurved in the Anaesthesiology.

Conculsion :

Similar studies and projects can be carried out with different Ayurvedic drugs and their efficacy and practical utility can be evaluated. The research field is very vast but if new generations come forward to carry out research work it will be possible for Ayurved to provide and even independent service system for relief of pain.

To conclude one can say that we must strive in future to give an even better and safer service of pain relief and care to our patients and if East and West meet, will provide the Best for Mankind.

[Reference : MUSING AYURVEDA 1992]
[International Ayurveda Conference]

Chapter : 13

Historical review of Indian Plastic Surgery

Late Dr. M. P. Yadwadkar

INTRODUCTION

The plastic surgery is the most recent surgical speciality accepted all over the world. It is supposed to be the very important to achieve high pro'eciency in this speciality. Plastic repairment has become a time demand for the present modern social culture especially in the Western advanced countries. And thus the advancement of the plastic surgery is fast.

The origin of the plastic surgery is India. It is a doubtless bold statement that we are the plunoer source of such a skilled and advance surgical speciality. India is the only who shares the lion part of the development and the practice the plastic surgery. One can trace back up to the time of the Ramayan wherein the reference is there that the transplantation of the lostles was successfully done by the Ashwinikumaras to lord Indra. (R 1)

India had the most civilised culture during these days of Ramayan when the rest of the World was just fumbling in the dark of the stone age. Still before Ramayan Lord Shivshankar also after a great war with his son unknowingly cut off his head and when he realised that, the implanted the elephant head on the body of his son. Thus he then was famous as lord Gajanan. To begin with anything with a holly spirit always heads to Lord Gajanan.

Sushrut Acharya

Irrespective to the mythological references in the recent harmy the famous Indian surgeon who is now very well accepted as father of Surgery in the World'. He was the first person on the earth who first wrote the scientific surgical contributions. Sushrutacharya was existing about 2000 years B.C. His surgical concepts were very Crystal clear and enough wide to include every modern surgical speciality. In his contribution Sushrutacharya has dealt a separate chapter on the plastic surgery - The title of the chapter is 'Karnabandha'. The basic principles, of the plastic surgery laid down by Sushrut are vertually unique and still stand for the test of the time. Thus it is doubtless that India was the first Country where the plastic Surgery was systematically practiced and was described. His surgical contribution is known as Sushrut Samhita.

Sushrutsanhita

Sushrutacharya has given a very brillient and mature contribution regarding the basic principles of the plastic surgery. A very disciplined classification of the plastic surgical techniques one can get in the Sanhita. It is really astonishing that in the absence of the technological assets and the advancement the way he had brilliently dealt the subject of the plastic surgery is really best and worth worshipping.

Plastic Surgery in Sushrutsanhita

The concept of the skin grult and the podical graft has been recently introduced in the modern surgery. The surgical specialty of the plastic surgery is a now born field of the modern surgery but Sushrutacharya described the same 2500 years age.

In the Sushrutsanhita firstly he described the conditions of availability of the part and the graft. (R 2) In which he clearly states the THREE MUSTS.

. The unasserted blood must not be present.

.. There must not be haemorrhagic tendency.

... There must not be the bloodlessness.

If these three or either of them is present the plastic surgeon is going to land on the troubles, in his results.

The complications of the plastic surgery are also mentioned in the sanhita. And according to the traditional systems of the medical practice in India, the basic physiological factors are the 'three doshas. 'They are supposed to be responsible for the production, existance and the distribution of the body eliments as well the life as a whole. Thus the complications of the plastic surgery are also based on these three doshas. They can be as follows :-

. Inflammation -- due to Pitta.

.. Suppuration -- due to Kapha.

... Pain -- due to Vat.

The Two Groups of Plastic Surgery

Sushrutacharya in his contribution on the plastic surgery has mentioned the two main groups.

. Sandhan karma : Repairative surgery

.. Vaikrutapaham : Cosmatic technique

In the repairative surgery, the Indian history of the plastic surgery includes only the Rhinoplasty, Auroplasty and the Labioplasty. There is no other reference of any other part indicative for the repairative surgical procedures. The reason being there was no timely demand for the other parts. It was the time during Sushrutacharya, that the Government used to adopt such a custom of the punishment in which the ears, nose and the lips were cut off. And it becomes very aquward for the person to be social and to mix up with masses. Thus the plastic repair of these parts had been an essential entity in the medical practice. But that was certainly a secret factor as would had against the govt. Rather plastic surgery was social crime during those days. But Sushrutacharya had made a bold step on the academic ground. He first time put forth the principles and the operative steps of the plastic surgical procedures, in the history of the plastic surgery.

The Repairative Surgery

There are three main repairative procedures pertaining to ear, nose and the lips.

(A) Auroplasty

Sushrutacharya has described various procedures of the repairative plastic surgery for the ear as per the deformity, and the tissue availability. If one carefully goes through the ancient Indian surgical text, it can be clearly understood that all the repairative plastic procedures can be grouped again in to three groups.

For the verticle deformities of ear lobule.

.. For the transverse deformities of ear lobule.

... For the irregular deformities of ear lobule.

For all of them the total procedures described are fifteen in the ancient Indian surgical text of the plastic surgery.

For the first group of the deformities the following are the procedures :

1. Nimisandhankar
2. Utapbhedak

3. Vallurak
4. Asangima
5. Gandakarna

Let the second group of the deformities the procedure described are as follows.

1. Aacharya
2. Kapatsandhik
3. Adhikapatsandhik
4. Nirvodham
5. Vyayogitam

For the third deformities though the names are enumerated the repairative procedures are not mentioned as it is strongly stated that these deformities are irrepairable and from the reputation point of view the surgeon should not deal with them. Those conditions are :

1. Sankshipta
2. Heenkarna
3. Yashtikarna
4. Valikarna
5. Kakashtak

The basic principles narrated in the Sushrut Sanhita from India about 2500 years ago. They are as follow about the Auroplasty.

1. Central Puncture for Elongated lobule :

To restore a normal neatly designed shape of the ear lobule and the pina in a case of a very small ear lobule, Sushrutacharya has adviced to puncture it the central region. Or even sometimes in the cartilage of the ear, and then ask the patient to wear the heavy rings. The weight of the rings should be gradually increased. This helps the pina and the lobule to get (R/3) elongated. No much operative interference is then needed.

2. Temporal-Parallal Incision for the Tissue availability

A parallel incision to the long axis of the pinna is made in the temporal region by the side of the lower pole of the ear and the skin is made available for the repairative procedure. (R/4)

3. Skin aligments according to defects

Sushrutacharya has very keenly guarded about skin approximations. In this aspect for the better plastic results he has adviced to consider the defects priest to the surgery. If the outer portion is longer, the future line should lie internally and vice-a-versa. (R/5)

4. Slidding Graft in Assemplasly

If the ear defect is like "Aasangima' of 'Gandhatna' in which the ear lobule is enough thick to one side and defective on the other side. Then the thick side is splitted in to two portions and the one portion is slided over the defective part for the repairative procedure. And thus the defective part is turned to a beautiful ear. (R/6)

5. Pedical Flap Graft

If the tissue of the defective ear lobule inadequate for the repairment, Sushrut states that a skillful surgeon under such circumstances takes a beautiful flap from the area of the cheakin-such a why that it remain; viable by the blood supply from the root. (R/7)

Rhinoplasty

This is a second variety of the repairative surgery we can find in the ancient Indian surgical texts. The description is in very brief but very meaningful and rhythumic too. (R/8)

The complete operative procedure of the rhinoplasty is described in the Sushrut Sanhita. This can be summarised as follows :

Take a leaf of any tree which has equal surface area as well the shape of the part of the nose to be repaired. Keep it on the cheak and markout the marqbins from all sides on the skin. The essential debridement of the defective area of the nose is done. Then the skin flap that is marked is dessected out with an uniform thickening and a root attachment for the maintenance of the vibility. Then this flap is impianted over the debrided are of the defective nose. Few necessary stiches are taken. Then the two hollow tubes are introduced in the nostrils and the wound is closed with a very clean (storlle) dressing of the cloth. The introduction of the two hollow tubes in the nostriles serve the dual purpose. The maintenance of the air-ways and the provision of the essential elivation of the nose for the natural texturisation of the particular area.

The most important and the interesting part one can note in the Indian history of the plastic surgery as far as the rhinoplasty is concerned that the whole operative procedure has never claimed to be complete in a single setting. Moreover Sushrutacharya emphasises that when the primary healing is about to complete again the necessary manuplations should be done. This is done by cutting or elevating the edges or some times the elevated edges are supressed down. For this multiple setting are said to be necessary.

LIBLOPLASTY :

In the historical texts of the Indian plastic surgery the surgeons who can perform the repairative surgery for the defective nose and the lips are expressed a great honour. The surgical procedure as such the thinopla sky resembles with that of the libloplasty too. The only difference is of the tubes in the nostriles.

The history of the plastic surgery has also taken the alert cognition of the famous reconstruction of Cowajee's nose by a native surgeon in Pune, Maharashtra. This was keenly observed by the two men of the East India Company. They were Mr. Cruso and Mr. James Findlay. When they returned home to England they published an article in 'Gentleman's Magazine'. The operative steps describd in this article are exactly similar to that of the steps described in Sushrut Sanhita.

Post operative

Some DON'TS are specifically mentioned in ancient Indian plastic surgical concepts for the better post-operative results. If they are not followed the results are bound to be hazardus. (R/8)

Rubbing of the repaired part, sleeping during the day time, exertion, heavy meals, sexual, inercourse, sun-bath or hot lomentation, too much speakings are the aspects to be avoided otherwise the results of the plastic repairs are certainly bad.

VAIKRUTAPAHAM

It is the cosmatic approach in the treatment of the scars and wounds. The scar may mismatch the healthy complex of the skin. The main procedures included in the aspect of the cosmatic approach known as the Vaikrutapaham, are intended towards the informative changes in healed ulcers, so that the scar should be developed in such a way that it will be perfectly matched to the rest of the complexion of the skin.

Following are the procedures described in the reformative surgery in the ancient Indian plastic surgery.

1. KRUSHNAKARMA

If the scar is leading to a white patch it should be

converted into the black colouration as per the complexion of the skin. This is called as Krisanakarma. (R/10)

2. PANDUKARMA

If the scar is Lending to blackness it should be converted into the fair whiteness. This is called as the Pandukarma. (R/11)

3. SAVARNIKARAN

If the skin developes the discolouration other than white or the black the procedure that is practiced is called as the Savarnikaran.

4. ROMSANJANAN

This is only Sushrutacharya's concept to stimulate the growth of the hair follicias as natural as on the rest of the skin over the area of the wound. Even in the modern concept this process is still not maturely looked after.

The reformative plastic surgical concepts are the best contributions from India in the history of the plastic surgery in the world. They are laid down first time in a very systematic and the scientific manner by the Great Acharya Sushrut 2500 years ago in India which are still equally truth like the computerised concepts of any other science.

REFERENCES

1. Shshrut Sanhita - Dr. Ghanekarshastri.
2. Dr. Deshpande and Sharma, 'Development of Plastic surgery in East and West', in Chikitcha Prasad, Aug. 1970.
3. History of Medicine - Dr. Numbergar.
4. Weber's History of the Medicine.
5. Marathi Charak Sanhita - Dr. P. H. Kulkarni (Sagar Prakashan) (1983)

[Reference : Deerghayu International, 1985]

Chapter : 14

Raktarsha & Mocharasa Yoga - a Study

VD. S. P. SARDESHMUKH
V. SHAILESH NADKARNI

Respected Chairman, Ayurvedic Scholars and Delegates.

In the next few minutes, I will be discussing before you a disease which is very commonly found in India these days, namely RAKTARSHA i.e. bleeding piles. We often come across so many patients when complain of per rectal bleeding off and on.

In such cases, often we find that the first goal that we have to achieve is to stop the per rectal bleeding as in most cases it is the all important pure blood i.e. जीव रक्त that is lost.

देहस्य रुधिरं मूलं रूधिरेव धार्यते।
तस्मात् यत्नेन संरक्ष्ये रक्तं जीव इति स्थिति:।।

सु. सु. १४/४४

To accomplish this objective, mocharasa, the niryasa or Gum of Shalmali (Bombax malabaricum) was used in the study being presented to you. The details of the drug administered will follow.

Let us in brief discuss the anatomical details of the part that is most visibly affected, i.e. the Rectum.

The Rectum is continuous with the pelvic colon (स्थुलान्त्यऽ प्रतिबद्धम्). While before it ends in the anal canal three lateral curves are also described. The upper one convex to the right, a middle one convex to the left and a lower convex to the right in front of the tip of the cocey.

The rectum is about 12 cm long. Besides these, there are certain permanent horizontal folds. There are usually three (3) of these horizontal folds of semilunar shape तस्मिन् वलयस्तिम: one is situated at the commencement of the rectum (प्रवाहणी) on the right side, the second extends inwards from the left side of the tube at a slightly lower level (विसर्जेनी) and third, the longest and most constant one projects backwards from the fore part of the rectum opposite the fundus of the urinary bladder (संवरणी). These folds are about 11 mm in width (एवं अंगुलोच्छिता) and contain some of the circular fibres of the gut. In an empty state the overlap each other. They use seems to be to support the weight of the faecal matter and prevent is urging towards the anus where its presence always excites a sensation demanding its discharge. The etiopathology of Raktarsha can simply be described in a sentence viz. the hot, spicy, heavy i.e. difficult to digest, viruddhahar, along with improper vihar such as improper sitting postures etc. are responsible for the Raktadushti and causing Raktarsha i.e. bledding piles.

But it would be proper at this stage for me to elaborate in a little more detail what these terms mean in today's life.

The eating habbits of man can be broadly classified into 3 catagories.

(1) To eat even when no apetite exists i.e. अन्यगन

(2) To overeat just because of over-hunger, i.e. अन्यगन

(3)To overeat sometimes and not to eat at all at other times. i.e. वियप्राशन

Basically it is the second catagory of habit which leads to lowering of the digestive power (i.e. मन्दाग्निता) and is the real cause of रक्तार्ग i.e. bleedings piles.

Hence the etiopathology of Raktarsha can be explained thus :

In a situation when the digestive power is quite lowered, if a person goes on consuming such foods like milk shakes and milk products, fast food products containing various preservatives, products prepared by using fermentation process etc. become responsible for pittavruddhi.

The blood or Raktadhatu which is the ashraya of pitta is a slightly alkaline substance having a pH of 7.4. In cases where pittavruddhi takes place, the pH is lowered resulting in the acidity of blood going up. This blood gets the required and all important in the and manifests itself in the form of bleeding.

गुरु मधुर

अग्निमांद्य → अत्याग्निमांद्य → विदग्धर्जीर्ण

अभिष्यन्दी

आहार सेवन

च. चि. १४/९

अत्युष्ण कटु, अम्ल त्ठवण,

विदाही, हरितगाकादि

क्रोध, चिंता वर्षा, शरद

रक्तार्ष ← पित्तज अर्ष ← विट्भेद ← पित्तवृद्धी

In the study we conducted, it was decided that this loss of नाविरक्त i.e. Frank blood that goes out of the body through the anus has to be prevented within 48 hrs.

The drug used was the gum of Bombax malabaricum in the form of ksheerpak. The method used for preparing the Ksheerpak was the one described by Late Yadavji Trikamji Acharya.

As per this preparation, 2 gms of podered gum of Bombax malabaricu i.e. मोचरस was mixed with 30 ml i.e. six tea spoonfuls of water and 6 teaspoonfuls of cow milk and heated till the water content of the mixture goes. The siddha ksheer was given twice a day to the patients of Raktarsha and their faces ere examined for fresh and/or occult blood. This examination as carried out for 48 hrs. to see the raktastambhak effect of the used preparation.

The entire study was based on the sootra

The data of the examined patients is a follows :

Total number of Raktarsha patients taken for study = 30.

DIVISION ACCORDING TO SEX

Males	16
Females	14

DIVISION ACCORDING TO AGE

12 to 30 years	4
31 to 45 years	20
46 to 60 years	4
61 and above	2

DIVISION ACCORDING TO SRAVA

Dry (Shushka)	0
Bleeding (Sravl)	30

DIVISION ACCORDING TO PERIOD OF SUFFERAGE

1 month to 12 months	12
1 year to 5 years	14
5 years and more	4

DIVISION ACCORDING TO NUMBER OF ARSHAS

Only one	12
Two	15
Three	03

DIVISION ACCORDING TO SENSATION AT THE TIME OF PASSAGE OF STOOL

Only pain	07
Only burning	08
No specific sensation	03
Little pain + Little burning	15

DIVISION ACCORDING TO BLEEDING PATTERN

(a)	i.	Prior to the passage of faeces	05
	ii.	Along with the faeces	01
	iii.	After the faeces	06
	iv.	Prior to & after the the passage of faeces	18
(b)	i.	Drop by drop	21
	ii.	Continuous flow	09
(c)	i.	Less	08
	ii.	Medium	11
	iii.	Excess	11

RESULT OBTAINED

100X cure 21 patients	70%
Remarkable improvement 03 patients	20%
Marginal improvement 06 patients	20%
No cure 00 patients	0%

[Reference : Deerghayu International : 1990]

Chapter : 15

Clinical trial on 169 patients Godhamajja Dahan Chikitsa in Kurup, corn cauterization with Godhamajja

Prof. R. B. Gogte

During practice especially in rural area development of curns on soles of the feet is very common condition. It produces pain while walking resulting in discomfort. Many times these corns are more than one.

The usual practice is to excise them under local or general anaesthesia and cauterize the raw wound with carbolic acid and suturing. Patient requires two or three dressings post operatively, is unable to walk well for two days postoperatively, spends half an hour for operative procedure. This results in abstinence from the duty, costs more to the patient for operative charges, medicines & post-operative dressings and still the chance of recurrences are possible in few patients.

As on Ayurvedic surgeon I gave a thought on the problem and decided to do cauterization with red hot iron shalaka using godamajja as sneha : <u>AFTER HAVING A FOLLOW UP FOR FIVE YEARS. I CAME TO THE CONCULUSION THAT IT WORKS WELL, RECURRENCE IS LESS, COSTS ONLY 2-3 RUPEES.</u>

NO DRESSINGS AND NO OBSTINENCE FROM THE DUTY.

(1)	Total patients treated	169	
	Followup after five years patients reported	86	
	No reporting	76	
	Letters return back	7	
(2)	Lowest age patient	3 years	
	Oldest patient	62	years
(3)	86 PATIENTS REPORTED		
	TOTAL RELIEF	4	56.9%
	Total relief with 2nd sitting	2	
	Relief regarding pain only	9	10.4%
	No relief	26	30.3%

KODAR (CORN) AS DIAGNOSED IN AYURVEDA

Usually there is a history of prick of thorn, nail, hard gravel or an irritation at a particular spot by pointed substances like nail of chapple, etc. Due to this irritation or a traum Tridoshas mainly Kapha & Wata develop changes in their gunas and produce Dhatu vaishammya in subcutaneous fat & vessels resulting into small triangular swelling with the point of a triangle towards shira. The common sites are sole of the foot, toes and rarely on palm.

शर्करोन्मथितेपादेक्षते वा कण्टकादिभि।
भेदोरक्तानुगेश्वेवदोपेर्वा जायते नृषाम्।
सकील कठिनो ग्रंथिर्निम्नध्योन्नतो पि वा।
कोल मात्रे सरुक स्त्रावो जायते कदरस्तु सः।। सु.नि.
१३/१०.११

हस्तयोः पादयोश्चापि गभिरानुगतं सरम्।
मांसकीलं जनयतः कुपितो कफमारूतो।। - मधुकोष
शर्करा घटकर्परसंडादयः हस्तयोरपीति भोजः।।

TREATMENT IN AYURVEDA

After doing the excision of the corn (kadar) encircle the excised area by dough of Masha.

Fill in the sneha in the ulcer and cauterize with red not Shalaka :

उत्कृत्य दग्ध्वा स्नेहेन जयेत कदरसंन्नकम्।
व्रणस्य परितो माएकत्केन दृढां पाती कृत्वा।
स्नेहनं तां पूरयित्वा दहेत्। इन्दु अ. स. उ. ३७

Instead of following the above technique I did little modification. The first part of excision was omitted. Godhamajja was applied over the corn without circling it with Mesha dough. Deep Dahanakarma was done by modified Jambostha Wadana Shalaka. Depth was decided by a sign "Loss of resistance produce by the corn." Adhesive plaster was applied on the Cauterize wound with out any sneha.

Initially vegitable fat in the form of DALDA was used but it was melting much earlier and the results were not promising and hence later on an Animal Fat Godhamajja was used as a sneha. The results were promising.

In the treatment no specific Shalaka has been described. LOHA SHALAKA WAS SELECTED IN RELATION TO MATERIALS DESCRIBED FOR DAHANKARMA IN CYSTS, GLANDS, TUMORS, ETC. AND PAIN RELIEVING PROPERTY IN RELATION WITH SKIN & SUBCUTANEOUS ADIPOSE TISSUE.

गेथ्यर्बुदर्शो भंगदरगंडमाला श्लीपदान्त्रवृद्धि दुष्टव्रण गतिनाडया गाढ पूयातकेषु जाम्बवोष्ठ सूची शलाका धृत गुडमधुच्छिष्ठ तैल वसा हेमताप्रोरूप्यकांस्यर्मास दाहः।।

अ.स.सू. ४०

अथेमानि दहनोपकरणनि भवति तद्यथा.........

पिप्यत्यजाशकृग्दोदंतशर शलाकाजांबवोष्ठेतर लोहाक्षोद्रगुडस्नेहाश्च।
तत्र पिप्यत्यजा शकृग्दोदंतशर शलाकास्त्वग्गतानां, जाम्बवोष्ठ तर लोहा मासगतानां क्षौद्रगुडस्नेहाः सिसस्नायुसंध्यास्थिग तासनाम। सु.सु. १२.४

त्वक् मांससंश्रितो वायुः त्वग्दाहैनैव शाम्यति।

Dahanakarma done on carns was of deep 'Bindu' type

तत वलय बिन्दु विलेमा प्रतिसारणमिती दहनविशेषाः

सु.स्. १२.४१

Actual procedure

1) The part was cleaned with water & dried completely.

2) Vasapinda was kept on the area of corn.

3) Dahankarma was done with red hot shalaka upto the depth "till resistance of the corn goes off.

4) Sticking plaster was applied directly an dagadha vrana.

No siddha ghrita or tail was applied

स्नेहदग्धे क्रियां स्क्षां विशेषेणवचारयेत्।।

सु.सू. १२.२७.२

Paschatkarma - Post Dahan chikitasa

1) Sticking plaster was removed on 4 to 6th day

2) No dressing

3) Those who had little signs of infammation were dressed with appropriate medicines.

4) In Asamyaka Daha recautaraisation was done.

5) Those who had little giddiness after dahan-cold water was sprinkled on the face of the patient c Ashawasan chikitasa.

Interrance of the work done

1) Relieves pain

2) Cost only 2-3 Rupees

3) No abstinence from the duty

4) No dressings

5) 56% cure rate + 4% second cauterization

6) 30% recurrance

7) 10% relief only in pain factor

[Reference : Deerghayu International : 1991]

Chapter : 16

Ayurvedic management of Accidental intra cerebral Haemorrhage

(A CASE REPORT)

DR. LAKHAPATI A.M., DR. G. S. LAVEKAR, DR. DALAL N.P.,

DR. DESHMUKHA R.D. & Resident

Doctors Government Ayruvedic College, Hospital Nagpur

In General, the surgical aspect of Ayurveda as always estimated under or neglected, in such circumstances one cannot think of emergency or treatment of serious conditions.

But surprisingly a case of accidental intracerebral haemorrhage is successfully treated with the Ayurvedic line of treatment, precise case report of the same is narrated here.

A 38 years old male patient was admitted to an allopathic teaching hospital, with following history.

Sudden onset of weakness in left extremities inability to speak clearly, inability to move the left extremities, incontinence of urine and defaecation, intense headache, irrelevant talk were present.

Necessary investigations were done, the findings of important investigations were as follows.

B.P. 210/140 mm. of Hg.

Funduscopy - Optic cups visible on both sides, Areterio venous nipping on left side.

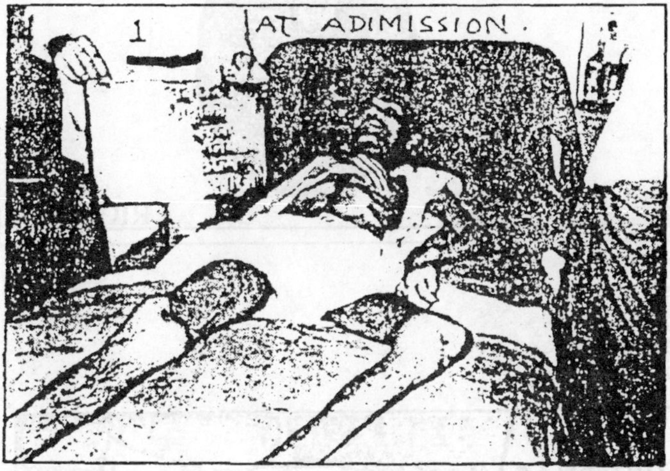

E.C.G. - WNL

CAT-SCAN - Haematoma in rt. thalamic and mid-brain region.

X-Ray - Skull - NAD

C.S.F. - Suger 87 Mg%, Chlorides 530 Mg%, Proteins 50 Mg% & Xynthochromic Lymphocytes - HPF.

Considering above findings the diagnosis was made as Moderate Hypertension with cerebravascular Empolism (Haemorrhagic) with Hemiparesis left.

The patient was treatment with standard line of treatment with, Drugs only, for twenty one days with no improvement inspite of this the patient was discharged

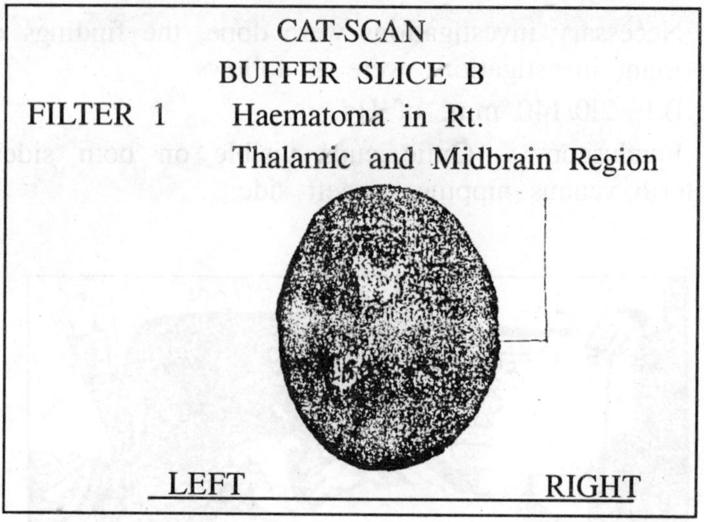

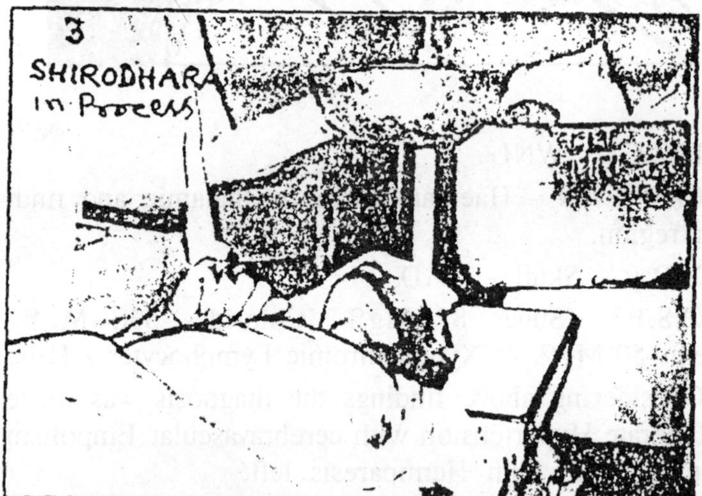

Shirodhara in Process

-- Oral Glycerol loz. T.D.S. % 4 days.

Tab. Aldomet 1 QID

Salt restricted diet

Physio theropy exercises

To come for review after 30 days.

The patients relatives thought to have the alternative Ayurvedic treatment. The patient was brought to the Shalya O.P.D. of Govt. Ayurvedic College Hosp., Nagpur for the treatment.

The patients was examined, the reports were observed and the patient was admitted in Shalya I.P.D. An understanding was given to the relatives about the prognosis (साध्या साध्यात्व) of the patient.

The details history was taken and revealed that the patient was regular drinker and after fall from the cycle he developed the left hemiporesis and other sign symptams for which he was brought to the Allopathic Medical College, Nagpur.

Again the patient was examined thoroughly in I.P.D. with Ayurvedic view. The following findings were present.

Left Hemiparesis. -- वामपक्ष कर्म हानी / वाम पक्ष वद्य

Aphasis. -- वाक्संग

Stool & Urine incontinence. -- मलमुत्र धारण अभाव

Headache.-- शिर:शूल

Insomnia. -- निद्रानाश

B.P. 150/120 mm of Hg. -- व्यानबल

Pulse 94/mm. -- नाडी

Pupils/BERL.-- कनिनिका

Apart of this the inpairment of optimum functions, of intelect (बुद्धि) and memory (स्मृती) was noted by lack of association to stimulii.

The location of Pathology (स्थान संक्रय) was revealed from the scan report i.e., Haematoma in Right thalamic and midbrain region.

As the lesion was in the Uttamanga (- मस्तिष्क) i.e., the intracerebral haematome (मस्तिष्कगत रक्त संचिती) was the main causative factor for the impairments of mainly the vatic functions.

The treatment was planned to evacuate the haematoma (मार्गावरोध) and to strengthen the affected parts of the body. The following line

At the time of Admission 12-4-88

-- Insomnia
-- Incontinence of stool and Urine
-- Aphasia
-- Loss of Memory to recognise the relatives.
-- Weakness of Lt. extremities and unable to stand. the stick for a short distance.
-- Flexion, Extention Movement sluguish
-- General debility
-- Body weight 34 kg.
-- Loss of Appetite
-- Headache
-- B. B. 160/120 mm / Hg
-- Hb 9.8% gm.

Improvement 15 days after treatment (27-4-88)

-- Sound sleep for 5 to 6 hours in the night.

-- Patient can recognise the sense of desire for micturation and defecation control over both the acts.

-- Indistinct but low pitch talk.

-- Can recollect many a things and able

-- Lt. extremities museles power regaine upto 3 + and patient was able to walk with

-- Movement improved.

-- Feeling energetic

-- 36 kgs.

-- Improved.

-- Absent

-- BP 140/90 mm / Hg.

-- Hb 11% gm.

of treatment was given.

– The patients scalp shaving was done and tap irrigation with medicated decoction i.e., Dashamoola kwatha was done prior to leach applications. (शिरोधारा)

– Anutail medicated nasal oil drops instillation (नस्य) was advocated once in a day for 15 days.

– Three leeaches were applied over both temporal regions on every alternate days, such ten seatings were given in each seating 15 to 20 cc. impure vitiated blood was removed.

– The powder of Glycereza Globra (यष्टी मधूचूर्ण) 2 gms. thrice in a day.

– The Sangeyasad bhasma (संगेयशद भस्म) 125 mg x twice in a day with honey.

– The Khamiregavjava, Ambari (खमिरेगावजवा, अंबरी) 5 gms. twice in a day.

– Saraswatarishta (सारस्वतारिष्ट) 15 ml. x twice in a day after food.

– Tab Aldoment 1 BD

– Bramhighrita (ब्राह्मी घृत) 15 ml. at bedtime.

– Apart to this daily whole body massage with Mahavatvyadhihar taila (महावात व्याधि हरतैल + अश्वगंधातैल (४० ml) + नारायणतैल (४० ml) कुक्कुटमांस तैल) (२० ml) followed with whole body steambath was given regularly for 30 days. With the above treatment, slowly but steadily the improvement was observed in the patient as compared with the initial conditions.

The same treatment was continued for another fifteen days. Except the doses of aldoment was adjusted as per the B.P. reading. The patient was recovered totally except general weakness.

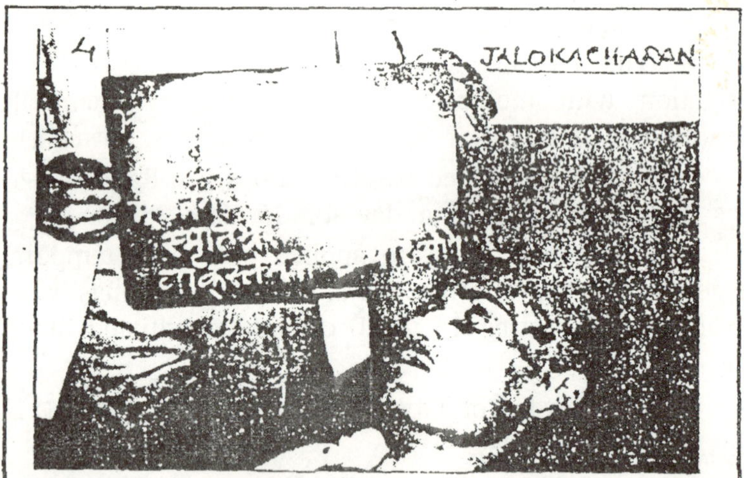

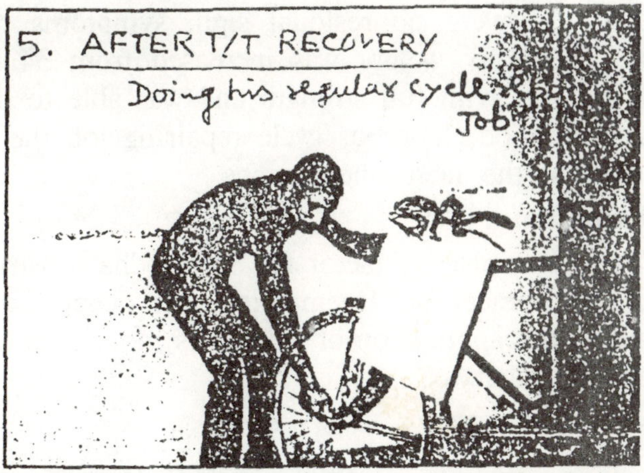

For further fitteen days the following treatment was continued.

– Whole body massage (सर्वांगर-नेहन स्वेदन) followed with steambath.

– Brahmighrita (ब्राह्मी धृत) 15 ml. at bed time.

– Anutail nasal drops (अणु तैल नस्य)

– Saraswatarishta (सारस्वतारिष्ट) 15 ml x twice daily.

– Shatavarikalpa (शतावरी कल्प) 15 gm. x twice daily with milk

– Tab aldoment 1/2 BD.

Thereafter, the patient was discharged with advising the following treatment, to be continued, for one month.

– Brahmighrita (ब्राह्मी घृत) 15 ml. at be time.

– Anutail drops (अणुतैल नस्य)

– Sharaswatarishta (सारस्वतारिष्ट) 15 ml. twice daily.

– Shatavarikalpa (शतावरी कल्प) 15 gm. x twice in a day with milk.

At the time of discharge the patient was totally

recovered therewere no residual sign. symptoms of the disease. The body weight was increased from 34 kg to 40 kg. He was with full strength and was able to do his routine livelihood, laborous cycle repairing job the same is evident in the later photographs.

Discussion :

The main causative factor for Srotorodha (obstructive lesion) was intracerabal Haematoma. For deeply situated haematoma the application of leeches is more effective as advised by Acharyas.

– अवगाठे जलौकस - सु. शा. ८/२५

– ग्रथितं जलजन्मभि - अवगाठे जलौकस / वा. सु० २६/१३

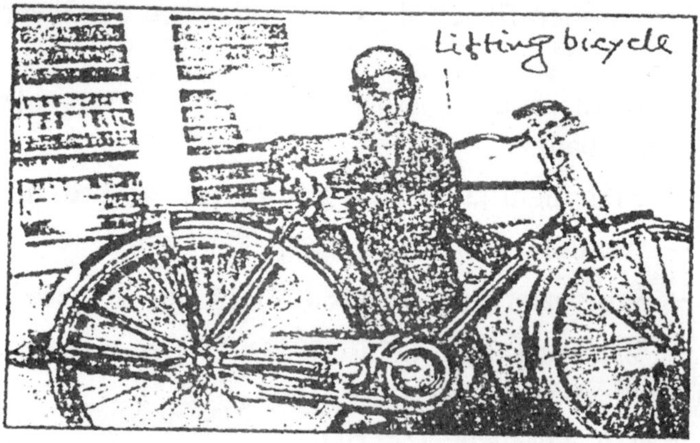

This selective Bio-blood aspiration has played an important role in clearing the Srotorodha (Obstructive Pathology)

– The tap irrigation of scale region (शिरोधारा) has helped to eliminate the diseased blood by increasing circulation of that region.

– The Khamiregavjava Ambari - The main active ingredient is Ambar which is an organic substance used in hemiplegia. It has got haematoma dissolving action.

– Yashatimadhu - Clycereza Elabra.

– This herbal drug is useful in reduing the inflamatory edema particularly that of haemorrhagic in origin.

– The sangeyashad Bhasma - is highly effective in the vitiated vata (neurogenic disordered) particularly that of Pakshavadha type disorders (Peresis). Apart to this it has got the property of abscrbing oedematous tissue fluid and thus releiving the tissue oedema.

– The Sarasvatarisha with Gold. This Elixir is an Excellent time tested remedy for insomnia impaired memory and other intelect associated disorders. it also improves the speech disorder.

– Mahavatvyadhihar taila - This oil is a mixture of Narayantial 40 ml. Asvagandha tail 40 ml. and Kukkutomamsa tails 20 ml. Regular massage of this oil followed with steam bath strengthening the muscle and thereby increasing muscle power.

– Bramhigruta - This mediated ghee is effective in loss of memory, headache and other related Psycho-smatic disorders.

This concise discussion clarified the modus operandii advocated in the above case.

This is a rare but successful example of serious condition treated with Ayurvedic line of treatment. Hope this will initiated to others to dare and act in similar conditions where other pathics are helpless.

[Reference : International Seminar 1996]

Chapter : 17

Evaluation of cosmetic value of Sneha Sutra and special Ointment in Surgical Wounds

DR. ABHAY HARISH PATHARE
-GUIDE-
DR. G. S. LAVEKAR
DIRECTOR
CENTRAL COUNCIL FOR RESEARCH IN AYURVEDA
& SIDDHA
NEW DELHI

INTRODUCTION

गण्डादुत्पाट्या मांसेन सानुबन्धेन जीवता।
कर्णपालीमपालेस्तु कुर्यान्निर्लिख्य शास्त्रवित्।।

– सु. सू. १७/२५

It is Sushruta who first successfully demonstrated the repair of the clipt earlobe with a patch of viable skin flap taken from the adjoining part. Sushruta's well known severed nose construction operation is called Indian Rhinoplasty and which is still in practice.

विश्लेषितायास्त्वथ नासिकाया, वक्ष्यामि सन्धानविधिं यथावत्।
नासाप्रमाणं पृथिवीरुहाणां, पत्रं गृहीत्वा त्ववलम्बि तस्य।।२७।।
.... समां च कुर्यादतिवृश्चमांसाम्।।३१।।

– सु. सू. १७

The important contribution of Sushruta, in plastic surgery is particularly that of transplantation of viable skin flaps. The art of reconstructing nose, ears, cleft lips has been well described in the Sushruta Samhita. Doctor Hirschbery of Berlin says, "The whole plastic surgery in Europe took a new flight when these cunning devices of Indian workmen became known to us".

It is interesting to note that in 17th Century the severed nose construction operation i.e. rhinoplasty was performed at Poona (Maharashtra State) on an Indian bullock cart person.

A Lightened Niranjan before the idol of god served as source of inspiration for using a similar sneha as a suturing material in the cosmetic procedures.

To improve the cosmetic appearance of the scar, surgeons are using highly specialized absorbable / non-absorbable skin suture material. These suture materials are very costly. It was thought over and to over come this problem a skin friendly suture material considering the Ayurvedic point of view was considered worth trying to have cost effective suture material in the form of sneha sutra, which fulfills most of the following conditions.

(A) If an ideal suture material could be created, it would be :

- All-purpose composed of material which could be used in any surgical procedure

  (the only variables being size and tensile strength).
- Sterile.
- Nonelectroyltic, aoncapillary, nonallergic, and non-carcinogenic.
- Nonferromagentic, as is the case with stainless steel sutures.

- Easy to handle.
- Minimally reactive in tissue and not predisposed to bacterial growth.
- Capable of holding securely when knotted without fraying or cutting.
- Resistant to shrinking in tissues.
- Absorbed with minimal tissue reaction after serving its purpose.

However, because the *idea* all-purpose suture does not yet exist, the surgeon must select a suture that is at least as close to the ideal as possible and maintain the following suture qualities :

1. High uniform tensile strength, permitting use of finer sizes.
2. Consistent uniform diameter.
3. Sterile.
4. Pliable for ease of handling and knot security.
5. Freedom from irritating substances or impurities for optimum tissue acceptance.
6. Predictable performance.

It seems that Sneha Sutra is capable to the above mentioned qualities of Ideal suture materiel.

B) Size and Tensite Strength Of Suture :

Size denotes the diameter of the suture material. The accepted Surgical practice is to use the smallest diameter suture that will adequately hold the mending wounded tissue. This practice minimizes trauma as the suture is passed through the tissue to affect closure. Suture size is stated numerically. The smaller the size, the less tensile strength the suture will have.

The tensile strength of the tissue to be mendca (its ability to withstand stress) predetermines the size and tensile strength of the suturing material the surgeon selects. The accepted rule is that the tensile strength of the suture need never exceed the tensile strength of the tissue. However, sutures should be at least as strong as normal tissue through which they are being placed. It the tissue reduces suture strength over time. The relative rates at which the suture loses strength and the wound gains strength are important. If the suture bilogically alters the healing process, these changes must also be understood.

(C) Monofilament vs. Multifilament Strands

Sutures are classified according to the number of strands of which they are comprised.

Monofilament Sutures –

Monofilament sutures are made of a single strand of material. Because of their simplifed structure, they encounter less resistance as they pass through tissue than multifilament suture material. They also resist harbouring organisms which may cause suture line infection. These characteristics make monofilament sutures well-suited to vascular surgery.

Monofilament sutures tie down easily. However, because of their construction, extreme care must be taken when handling and typing these sutures. Crushing or crimping of this suture type can nick or create a weak spot in the strand. This may result in suture breakage.

Multifilament Sutures –

Multifilament Sutures consist of several filaments, or strands, twisted or braided together. This affords greater tensile strength, pliability, and flexibility. Multifilament sutures may also be coated to help them pass relatively smoothly through tissue and enhance handling characteristics. Coated multifilament sutures are well-suited to intestinal procedures.

(D) Absorbable and Non absorbable materials :

Suture materials are also classified according to their properities which enables them to get absorbed in the system. At the same time application of an Ayurvedic ointment which might help to accelerate the cosmetic appearance by reducing morbidity of the resultant scar is also one of the aims of this scientific study.

MATERIAL AND METHOD

To study the cosmetic results it was decided to use this suturing material (Sneha Sutra) on the facial incisions taken for cosmetic procedures, but in view of the senior teachers such type of study was being done for the first time, its positive or negative results were yet unknown. So, as a precautionary measure it was therefore decided to do the basic study on the hidden surgical incisions and that too on the incision of one direction. As a result this technique was used on abdominal incision preferably on inguinal hernia operations and appendicectomy operations, which will fulfill the idea of hidden surgical incision and of one directional incision i.e. oblique incision.

: Material :

The patients admitted in Shalya Department of M.A. Podar Hospital have formed an important clinical material. The patients undertaken for clinical study have following criteria :

A. Inclusion

1. Patient > 18 years and < 60 years
2. Hb% > 10 gm
3. Normal bleeding time and clothing time
4. Oblique abdominal incision i.e. preferably inguinal incision

B. Exclusion

The patients having following diseases were excluded from the study.

Anaemia (Hb% < 10 gm.), Diabetes mellitus, Jaundice,Cancer, Skin diseases, patients taking steriods and Immuno compromised patients.

Preparation of "Seneha Sutra"

Madura Coats 'Griffin' Cotton thread No. 10 was taken and cut into pieces of 9 inches each and then they were soaked in 'Go Ghruta' for 7 days. After that they were transferred in sterile box. Before use they were sterilizied along with the same box.

• For Skin suturing No. 18 half circle triangular needle was used.

• Sushruta has described the Rhinoplasty operation. During this procedure he has used different churnas to sprinkle on the would. The same churnas have been used in the preparation of an ointment with Go Ghruta as a base.

• Ingredients of special ointment :

1. Patang (Caesalpinia sappan)
2. Yastimadhu (Glycyrrhiza glabra)
3. Rasanjan (Prepared from Daru Haridra i.e. Berberis Aristata)

• For dressing 'Tegaderm' - A transparent dressing material was used.

• प्रोन्नम्य चैनामवचूर्णयेतु, पतङ्गयष्टीमधुकाञ्जनैश्च।।

– सु. सू. १६/२९

: Methodology :

Patients were selected as per the criteria of exclusion and inclusion. The scientific study was performed in Four Groups.

Group A

Pre operative 3 consecutive days Snehan and Swedan at the site of the operation followed by routine operative procedure with suturing by simple cotton thread.

This group consisted of 10 patients.

Group B.

Pre operative 3 consecutive days Snehan and Swedan at the site of the operation followed by special suturing i.e. Sneha Sutra.

This Group consisted of 10 patients.

Group C.

Two subgroups were made consisting of 7 patients in each.

In these groups no pre oleation (Snehan) and sudation (Swedan) had advocated.

C.1. In 7 patients the half medial part of the operative wound were sutured by Sneha Sutra and Lateral half were sutured by simple cotton thread.

C.2. In 7 patients medial half were sutured by simple cotton thread and Lateral half sutured by Sneha Sutra.

Group D.

Two subgroups were made consisting of 10 patients in each.

D.1. Pre operative 3 days Snehan and Swedan at the site of the operation followed by routine operative procedure with suturing by simple cotton thread and application of special ointment.

D.2. Pre operative 3 days Snehan and Swedan at the site of the operation followed by routine operative procedure with suturing by Sneha Sutra and application of special ointment.

Along with Subcuticular absorbable catgut sutures, interrupted type of skin sutures were taken and Tegaderm dressing applied for 7 days without change. Through this transparent dressing observations were noted on 3rd, 5th and 7th day respectively. Stitches were removed on 7th day and further observations were noted on 14th, 21st and 28th days respectively. The observations were taken in the following pattern.

*** OBSERVATION ***

Observations of the Surgical wound after suturing was done on 3rd, 5th & 7th day.

In follow up period observations were done on every 7th day of three consecutive weeks

CRITERIA OF OBSERVATION

	3rd Day	5th Day	7th Day
Discharge			
Swelling			
Redness			
Tenderness			
Pain			

CRITERIA OF OBSERVATION IN FOLLOW UP PERIOD

	14th Day	21st Day	28th Day
Appearance of the Scar			
Hypertropy			
Pain			
Surface			

OBSERVATION OF POST-APPLICATION OF OINTMENT

Spread	
Staining	
Irritation	

Properties of GHRUTA as mentioned in Treatise

GUNA : Guru, Snighdha. RASA : Madhur

VIRYA : Sheeta VIPAK : Madhur

Dosha-Karma : Vata-Pitta Shamak

Clinical Uses :

घृतं पित्तानिलहरं रसशुक्रौजसां हितम्।
निर्वापणं मृदुकरं स्वरवर्णप्रसादनम्।।

—च. सू. १३/१४

It reduces pitta and vata, useful for Rasa, Shukra and Oja, reduces burning sensation, Smoothens skin texture, improves the skin complexion and improves the quality of voice.

It is also medhya, dipaniya, rhidhya, vrishya, garbhasthapak, jwaraghna, balya, bruhaniya, rasayana, chakshushya and *vrana ropak* in nature.

सर्पिस्तैलं वसा मज्जा सर्वस्नेहोत्तमा मताः।
एषु चैवोत्तमं सर्पिः संस्कारस्यानुवर्तनात्।।

—च. सू. १३/१३

In Ayurveda four types of Sneha (fats) are described viz. Ghruta, Tail, Vasa, Majja. Baring tail all are of animal origin. Ghruta is the best amongst all of them because it shows a property like संस्कारस्यानुवर्तनात् - It not only maintains its original characteristics even after blending and heating with some other substances but also maintains the characteristics of that substance along with its own. It is also yogavahi in nature mean after mixing with a substance enhances the properties of that substance.

PROPERTIES OF *BERBERIS ARISTATA* as mentioned in Tretise

GUNA : Laghu, Ruksha RASA : Tikta, Kashaya

VIPAK : Katu VIRYA : Ushna

Clinical Uses :

Shothaher, Vedanasthapan, Vranashodhan, Vranaropak, Chakshushya, Varnya, Swedjanan.

❖ Preparation of *RASANJAN* :

Parts of roots of Berberis Aristata is boiled with water (water taken is 16 times the weight of the roots), when 1/4th of this total quantity remains it is filtered. To this decoction equal quantity of goat's milk is mixed and this mixture is again heated on a low flame, until it thickens This final thick product is *RASANJAN*.

❖ दार्वीक्वाथसमं क्षीरं पादं पक्त्वा यदा घनम्। तदा रसाञ्जनं ख्यातं नेत्रयोः परमं हितम्।।

रसाञ्जनं कटु श्लेष्मविषनेत्रविकारनुत्। उष्णं रसायणं दिक्तं छेदनं व्रणदोषकत।।

– भावप्रकाश

PROPERTIES OF *CASESALPINIA SAPPAN Linn.* as mentioned in Tretise

GUNA : Ruksha RASA : Kashay, Tikta, Madhur

VIPAK : Katu VIRYA : Sheet

DOSHA KARMA – Kapha-Pitta shamak

Clinical Uses :

In external application it acts as Vrana-ropak,

Raktastambhak, Kushtaghna. Decoction is used orally in internal hemorrhage.

In Dhanwantari and Rajnighantu it is described as KUCHANDAN

कुचन्दनं तु तिक्त स्यात् सुगन्धि व्रणरोपणम्

– धन्वतरी निघण्टु

पतंगं मधुरं शीतं पित्तश्लेष्मव्रणास्त्रनुत्। हरिचन्दनवद् वेधं विशेषाद् टाहनाशनम्।।

– भावप्रकाश

PROPERTIES OF *GLYCYRRHIZA GLABRA* as mentioned in Tretise

GUNA : Guru, Snigdha. RASA : Madhura.

VEERYA : Sheeta VIPAKA : Madhura

DOSHA : Tridoshahara

KARMA : Vrishya, Chakshushya, Vranaropak, Varnakar, Kanthya, Rochana, Kasshwasahara.

Clinicial Uses :

In Ayurveda it is used extensively as a demulcent, mild expectorant and anti-inflammatory agent. It relieves 'vata' and 'kapha' inflammation, it is also used in eye diseases, throat infections, symptomatic relief in peptic ulcer and as an antiarthritic agent.

या वेदना शास्त्रनिपातजाता तीव्रा शरीरम् प्रदुनोती जन्तोः।
घृतेन सा शान्तिमुपैति सिक्ता कोण्णेन यष्टीमधुकान्वितेन।।

– सु. सू. ५

व्रणशोथविषच्छर्दितृष्णाम्लानिक्षयापहा।

– भावप्रकाश

OBSERVATIONS AND RESULTS

The capacity to sustain strain of the suturing material is also important which is called as tensile strength. As it is desired that the sutured wound should heal properly without or very minimal scar and without sepsis, different suture materials are used to strengthen these suturing materials. They are made multi filamental or breaded or they are treated with different chemicals. These procedures are not free from the danger of sepsis in multi filamental threads or an unwanted allergic reaction to chemically treated threads. Hence there is always a need of universal tissue friendly suture material especially in the cosmetic surgical field.

To achieve this goal a multi filamental breaded cotton thread was treated with Go Ghruta. It is well known and well accepted fact that the ghruta resists biological growths hence is not perishable. Considering this property along with its healing properties ancient Acharyas were using Puran Ghruta before dressing the wounds. It also easily penetrates in the potential spaces. Considering these properties of the "Go Ghruta" the suturing material was diped in to melted Go Ghruta for 7 days.

To understand and to prove the above claims the tensile strength of the cotton thread and processed Sneha Sutra were studied and compared : so also in vitro studies of bacteriological growth were carried out. The results of the above studies are as follow :

No. 10 cotton thread is generally used to suture the skin of the surgical incision taken for hernia in the M.A. Podar Hospital.

This same thread marketed by Madura Coats Company was used to prepare Sneha Sutra. The purpose of the study was to find out whether the tensile strength of the thread changes due to its processing with Go Gruta, 10 samples of equal length of each of the thread i.e. simple cotton thread and the thread used to prepare Sneha Sutra of 1 month and 1 year 4 months age were taken from the same thread recl. These 10 unprocessed and 10 processed samples were subjected to study their tensile strength at V.J.T.I. Textile Department, Matunga, Mumbai. The result are tabulated.

TENSILE STRENGTH

& % BREAKING ELONGATION OF MEDICATED SURGICAL THREAD (SNESHA SUTRA)

PERFORMED ON 16TH APRIL, 2001 AT V.J.T.I. TEXTILE MANUFACTURER DEPT.

COTTON THREAD NO. 10 ORIGINAL Madura Coats Griffin

No.	TENSILE STRENGTH KG.	BREAKING EXTENSION CM.	% BREAKING ELONGATION
1.	2.650	0.9	18
2.	2.700	0.8	16
3.	2.350	0.9	18
4.	2,600	0.8	16
5.	2.050	0.8	16
6.	2.600	0.9	18
7.	2.750	1.0	20
8.	2.525	0.8	16
9.	2.475	0.8	16
10.	2.750	0.8	16
TOTAL	25.450	8.5	170
MEAN	2.545	0.85	17

* TENSILE STRENGTH =2.545 KG.

* BREAKING EXTENSION =0.85 CM.

* % BREAKING ELONGATION =17%

STANDARD DEVIATION**CO-EFFICIENT OF VARIATION

A	TENSILE STRENGTH	0.2033469	0.0799005
B	BREAKING EXTENSION	0.067082	0.07892
C	% OF ELONFATION	1.3416408	0.07892

FULL SCALE LOAD = 5 KG CROSSHEAD SPEED = 10 CM/MIN

CHART SPEED = 10 CM/MIN GAUGE LENGTH = 5 CM

TENSILE STRENGTH

& % BREAKING ELONGATION OF MEDICATED SURGICAL THREAD (SNESHA SUTRA)

PERFORMED ON 16TH APRIL, 2001 AT V.J.T.I. TEXTILE MANUFACTURER DEPT.

SNEHA SUTRA NO. 10 MEDICATED - ONE MONTH OLD

Madura Coats Griffin - Cotton Thread

No.	TENSILE STRENGTH KG.	BREAKING EXTENSION CM.	% BREAKING ELONGATION
1.	2.650	0.8	16
2.	2.625	0.9	18
3.	2.275	0.8	16
4.	2.500	0.8	16
5.	2.600	0.9	18
6.	2.575	0.9	18
7.	2.650	0.8	16

8.	2.250	0.8	16
9.	2.525	0.8	16
10.	2.250	0.8	16
TOTAL	24.900	8.3	166
MEAN	2.490	0.83	16.6

* TENSILE STRENGTH = 2.490 KG.
* BREAKING EXTENSION = 0.83 CM.
* % BREAKING ELONGATION = 16.6%

STANDARD DEVIATION**CO-EFFICIENT OF VARIATION

A	TENSILE STRENGTH	0.1585	0.0636546
B	BREAKING EXTENSION	0.0458	0.0551807
C	% OF ELONGATION	0.9165	0.0552108

FULL SCALE LOAD = 5 KG CROSS-
HEAD SPEED = 10 CM/MIN
CHART SPEED = 10 CM/MIN
GAUGE LENGTH = 5 CM

TENSILE STRENGTH

& % BREAKING ELONGATION OF MEDICATED SURGICAL THREAD (SNESHA SUTRA)

PERFORMED ON 16TH APRIL, 2001 AT V.J.T.I. TEXTILE MANUFACTURER DEPT.

SNEHA SUTRA NO. 10 MEDICATED - ONE MONTH OLD

Madura Coats Griffin - Cotton Thread

No.	TENSILE STRENGTH KG.	BREAKING EXTENSION CM.	% BREAKING ELONGATION
1.	1.275	0.8	16

2.	1.275	0.8	16
3.	1.250	0.6	12
4.	0.950	0.5	10
5.	1.325	0.6	12
6.	1.050	0.5	10
7.	1.200	0.6	12
8.	1.125	0.6	12
9.	1.250	0.6	12
10.	1.050	0.6	12
TOTAL	11.750	6.2	124
MEAN	1.175	0.62	12.4

*** TENSILE STRENGTH = 1.175 KG.**

*** BREAKING EXTENSION = 0.62 CM.**

*** % BREAKING ELONGATION= 12.4%**

*STANDARD DEVIATION**CO-EFFICIENT OF VARIATION*		
A TENSILE STRENGTH	0.11772921	0.100195
B BREAKING EXTENSION	0.0979795	0.1580314
C % OF ELONGATION	1.9595918	0.1580316

FULL SCALE LOAD = 5 KG CROSS-HEAD SPEED = 10 CM/MIN

CHART SPEED = 10 CM/MIN

GAUGE LENGTH = 5 CM

As the durability of the processed thread was studied along with that the bacteriological studies were also under taken for the Sneha Sutra and ointment to find out the growth of 5 usually found pathogenic bacterias in surgical wounds in vitro. The study was performed at Radhibai Watumal Hospital's Microbiology department, Mahim - Mumbai.

This study was done to find the effect of ointment

and Sneha Sutra (Medicated thread) on the bacteria usually infecting the surgical wounds by using pure cultures of the suspected organisms. The chart is self explanatory.

RADHIBAI WATUMULL GLOBAL HOSPTIAL

120, Veer Savarkar Marg, Mahim, Mumbai - 400 016

Tel. : 24453942, 24449968, 24446614

Date : 07-05-2001

Antibacterial properties of the given medicated threads (Sneha Sutra)

1) New thread (one month old) 2) Old thread one year one month old) & the Ointments were studied by diffusion assay

The Study was done on 5 specific organisms.

The sensitivity pattern was interpreted after 24 hrs. 48 hrs. & 72 hrs. of incubation.

. The inhibition zone was measured in mm & noinhibition was indicated as NI.

Organism		New Thread	Old Thread	Ointment
Staphylococcus	24 hrs.	1 mm.	1 mm.	2 mm.
–aureus	48 hrs.	1 mm.	2 mm.	2 mm.
	72 hrs.	1 mm.	2 mm.	2 mm.
Escherichia Coli	24 hrs.	NI	0.5 mm..	NI
	48 hrs.	NI	0.5 mm.	NI
	72 hrs.	NI	0.5 mm.	NI
Pseudomonas	24 hrs.	NI	NI	NI
	48 hrs.	NI	NI	NI
	72 hrs.	NI	NI	NI
Klebsiella	24 hrs.	1 mm.	2 mm.	1 mm.
	48 hrs.	1 mm.	2 mm.	1 mm.
	72 hrs.	1 mm.	2 mm.	1 mm.

Streptococcus pyogenus	24 hrs.	1 mm.	1 mm.	2 mm.
	48 hrs.	1 mm.	1 mm.	2 mm.
	72 hrs.	1 mm.	1 mm.	2 mm.

CONCLUSION

Considering the Observations and the Results of the study, following conclusions can be drawn.

(1)There is no significant change in tensile strength of sneha sutra of one month age in comparison to cotton thread of same gaze. However the tensile strength of the sneha sutra reduces as it grows older. Hence it would be worth while to find out its expiry date, this part is left for future study.

(2)In invitro studies it was observed that the sneha sutra prepared with Go Ghruta inhibits the growth of organisms which are frequently pathogenic in the surgical wound such as *Staphylococus aureus, Streptococcus Pyogenus, Pseudomonas, E. Coli, Klebsiella.* The area of inhibition is significant. Hence it can be concluded that the sneha sutra is capable of preventing the infection and in turn prevents suppuration caused by it.

(3)After the studies done on antibacterial properties of New Thread i.e. 1 month old Ghruta and Old Thread i.e. 1 year 1 month old Ghruta, the results showed that old ghruta exhibits more antibacterial properties than that by new ghruta. This result leaves a further ground for new researchers to use puran ghruta instead of new ghruta in preparation of Sneha Surta and observe the results.

It is interesting to note that all the Acharyas equivocally advocate Puran ghruta for better healing of wound.

(4)It was also observed that the ointment specially prepared for the study also inhibits the bacterial growth in the petridish (Media used - Nutrient Agar and MacConkey's Agar)

(5)It seems that the wound healing in the patients whose surgical wounds were sutured by sneha sutra was uneventful and the resultant scar is minimum as compared to traditional cotton thread. It was also noted that the suture marks were not that significant after 7th day, on macroscopic eye scrutiny. The scar of, sneha sutra sutured patients, was very similar to the adjacent skin up to the 28th day of operation, making it a significant cosmetic value.

(6)Patients where sutures were taken with sneha sutra and the dressing was done with application ointment did not show significant added effect as compared to patients sutured only by sneha sutra. However it was noted that the colour of the scar resembles to the adjacent skin after about two weeks from removing the sutures. It seems that the probable colouring property of one of the ingredients of the ointment viz. Patang (Caesalpinnia sappan) might be responsible for this effect, as this plant has colouring effect : hence it is widely used in textile industry.

(7)It is interesting to note that a group of patients were divided in equal groups and their wounds were sutured with sneha sutra medially and cotton thread laterally in the same patients in one group (i.e. group C1) and vise versa in the other group (i.e. Group C2). The findings were similar as seen in the conclusion drawn in No. 5 in this chapter. Hence it can be concluded that even in self controlled study sneha sutra has significant cosmetic effect as compared to cotton thread.

(8)Sneha Sutra is an ideal suture material for cosmetic purpose because of the following characteristics found during this study :

(a) Knot security without fraying or cutting

(b) Easy tissue passage.

(c) No skin allergic reactions.

(d) Tensile strength remains unchanged for one month.

(e) Not predisposed to bacterial growth.

Thought it was thought that to find out cosmetic effect of the materials under study an the facni scars it was then decided that since there are no clinical studies to guide, it would be worth while to study the effect of sneha sutra and ointment in the surgical wounds of oblique nature viz. surgical wound of Inguinal Hernia operation : which are usually hidden. We are aware that there are so many groups in this study and the sample size in each group is small. This study would be guide for further researchers to plan studies with larger sample size. As there are definite positive findings on the cosmetic effects of healing, scientific fraternity will be tempted to study the subject further.

BIBLIOGRAPHY

Sr. No.	Name	Author	Publisher
1.	Dravyaguna-Vigyan	Prof. P. V. Sharma	Chaukhambha Orientalia Varanasi (India) 1978
2.	Charak Samhita	AGNIVESA Revised by Charaka and Drudhabala	Chaukhambha Orientalia Varanasi (India) 1979
3.	Sushruta Samhita Sharir Sthanam	Dr.B.G. Ghanekar	Meharchand Lachamandas New Delhi 1978

4.	Sarth Sushruta Samhita	Vaidyraj Datto Ballal Borkar	Raghuvanshi Prakashan Pune
5.	ABC of plastic and reconstructive Surgery	Dai Davies	British Medical Journal 1985
6.	Fundamental Techniques of plastic Surgery and their Surgical applications	IAN A. McGREGOR Alan D. McGREGOR	Churchill Livingstone 19th Edition 1995
7.	Surgical Dressings and Wound Healing	Edited by K.J. Harkiss	Bradford University Press and Crosby Lockwood and Son. Ltd. - London
8.	Surgical Nursing	Colin Torrance Eue Serginson	Bailliere Tindall - London 12th Edition
9.	Applications of Biomaterials in Facial and Plastic Surgery	Editor Alvin I. Glasgold Frederik H. Silver	CRC Press - Boston
10.	ETHICON Wound Closure Manual		Division of Johnson & Johnson Ltd.

[Reference : Gold Medal Reciepient at International meet on evidence Based Ayurveda in daily practice, Pune, 20th August 2006]

Chaper : 18

A review of 45 (forty five) cases of Fistula in ano,

Treated by 'Ksharasutra' Made by Papaya latex

Dr. S. Dattatreya Rao
Tirupati, Andhra Pradesh, India.

INTRODUCTION

In Ayurvedic Surgery, the four fold approach to every disease would fulfill all the needs of surgeon. They are Kshara, Agni, Shastra Karmas and Rakta Mokshana. The kshara karma is most important, since it is less hazardous and can be useful in both the routs, the 'Antah parimarjana' and the 'Bahi Parimarjana' i.e. internal and external use. It is also used both as Medicine and Surgical measure. Kshara Sutra is a thread impregnated with the kshara, i.e. the alkaline powder of plant origin. By its properties the Kshara acts on the local tissue as chemical cautery, it scraps the tissue out and gives room for formation of healing tissue.

The ksharasutra is mentioned in all the Brihad Trayee, the 'charak samhita' the 'sushruta samhita'and the 'Ashtanga Hridaya'. But a detailed methodology is not mentioned. In later workes like Bhava prakasha also it found its place and was inpractise since ages in India But some how the actual usage of this method laid only with the traditional surgeons spreading across India.

The poineer work done by P. J. Deshpande et el., has created a new avenue for the surgeons to use this 'kshara sutra' in the diseases like fistula in ano. Since than a detailed methodology and scientific approach to the preparation and application of this thread has came into existance.

The use of kshara sutra is well appreciated in the field of surgery on fistula in ano besides in few other diseases. Because of the draw backs in conventional surgery over fistual in ano like recurrence, incontinence etc, this method is well accepted.

By the use of Ksharasutra in the fistula in ano the fistulous tract get scraped, cut through on the one hand and heal on the other hand. The process go on is stages for a long period. Because of the cauterization effect of the material used in the preparations, pain and discomfort troughout the regimen is a important point here both surgeon and patient worries.

The kshara sutra is made by the application of a kshara, the alkaline powder, to a thread with the help of latex expressed from a plant. The turmeric powder is also added to the this mixture to make it more potent. The conventional material used are found to be corresive and cause buring sensation, pain and imflamation in the tissue. The pain will be untolerable to the patient in few cases. Secondly the long period that is required to complete the procedure is a problem before the surgeon. So a quest is countinuing to prepare a thread which minimise the pain and reduces the length of period required for the treatment.

Keeping in view of the above problems search has been made to choose a material which can be used to prepare the kshara sutra and by which the pain component and the time factor are reduced.

The latex of papaya furit is considered here is his study with the use of Tankan Kshara as alkaline powders. The turmeric powder, (Haridra) is used asusual. The powder and latex mixed together and applied to the tread found to be very effective and the problems of pain and long period of treatment came down considerably along with usual advantages on non recurrences. A review of 45 cases is given below.

MATERIALS AND METHODS :

1. Kshara Sutra :

A. Material used :

a. Latex : The latex extracted from the tender fruit of Papaya (C-papaya linn).

b. The alkali : Taukan kshara (Tanken Bhasma) is used in this study.

c. Trumeric Powder : The powder of rhi zome of (curcuma - longa) is used to prepare the thread.

B. Drug - review.

a. Papaya is known as carica-papay and as Ernada karkati in sanskrit. The latex of fruit contains papaya it clots the milk due to the presence of milk curdling enzyme. In action this latex is similar to pepsin which digests the protiens, externally if used it removes papillary eruption. It also contains albuminiods.

b. Curcuma longa - is known as Haridra, the rhizome of the plant is used. It is widely used in domestic peparations and medicinal preperations It is well known aseptic and anti inflamatory agent. Its anti inflamatory action against histamine, egg albumin is well proved. There is a volatile oil present in it, called as curcumin with is soluble in alchohol. Its formula is C_{21} H_{20} C_6 the volatile acid is also termed as Turmeric oil.

c. Tankan Powder : Tankan Bhasma is also known as Tankan Kshara. Its composition is. It is alkalin in nature. It is useful as Kshara and as external application in many diseases.

C. **PH Values** : The pH values of all the ingrediants measured with the help of glass electrode and pH metre and corelated with the measurement obtained by pH paper method. The pH of the all the ingrediants, measured every time the thread is prepared. The pH value of the total mixture was also measured before application on the thread and recorded.

2. Kshara Sutra Preperation :

a. 20 No. cotton thread is used for preperation of thread since it has found to have enough tensile strength.

b. Kshara Sutra cabinet : For the preperation of Kshara Sutra, a box designed specially for the preperation of the thread is used. Which got stands to hold the thread, Fans for drying purpose and Uv. lamp for sterilisation. Strict aseptic precautions were also observed while preperation.

c. Application of Kshara : The thread is tightly fixed to the stands and the mixture of latex, tankan and haridra powder prepared and smeared on the thread for 10 times, each smear after the drying up of the earlier smear. Thus the formed tubes and sealed for use only when required. Thus 10 batches of threads were made in this entire study.

3. **The Clinical Plan :** It was decided to carry out the trial on all the patients two attended O.P. seeking relief from fistula in ano. These patients were well informed about the study and regimes they have to follow.

a. Types : All the types of Bhangandars except the Shataponka were included in the study as per the anatomical classificaton the anorectal, high and low anal sub mucus or subcutaneous veraties were considered. The multiple fistulas, and those which were along with other systemic problems were excluded.

b. Records : Specially prepared cards were used to record the particulars of the patients in detail each patients vital data is recorded, the chronicity of the case, the number of recurrences if any were considered.

c. Method of Application to Thread :

The Patients were prepared and made in lithotony position and thoroughly probed. In few cases fistulograms were also taken. Then with a meleable probe the probing was done and the internal opening is felt. Thus with the help of its eye the thread is applied.

The change of thread is done at weekly interval and this was carried out by the road and rail technique.

d. Follow up : The patients were asked to follow strict plans of follow up. So as to attend the clinics every week during the regimen and every month after the treatment of six monts and once in every 3 months than afterwards. The operated area was checked up each time particularly to rule out any chance of recurrence.

e. Estimation of unit cutting time (UCT)

As per the standard procedure the length of fistula was calculated by the length of kshara sutra applied in the beginning. (Deshpande., etal.) Than the unit cutting time was calculated with following principle and recorded. However the lengths of subsequent threads were also measured whenever a the new thread was applied.

The length of fistulae is the major factor for the progress the treatment and to estimate the cutting capacity of thread.

Formula : Unit cutting time

$$(UCT) = \frac{\textit{Total Number of days}}{\textit{Initial length in cm. of fistulae.}}$$

RESULTS AND DISCUSSION

As per the foresaid procedure Total of 45 patients studied with the use of Kshara Sutra made up of Papaya latex. The study was at random and open clinical trial. The patients were supplied with the O.P. cards indicating their registered number and other details.

1. SEX DISTRIBUTION :

There were 6 female cases in total of forty five cases. Thus only in 13.33% of patients were female which points out at low rate of incidence in females.

2. AGE DISTRIBUTION.

The youngest patient in male was of 16 years old and the oldest was 60 years. In females the patients were between 21 years to 40 years of age. (Table 1).

Table : 1 Sex and Age distribution :

Age groups	Male	Female	Total
11-20	4	1	5
21-30	12	2	14
31-40	10	2	12
41-50	9	1	10
51-60	4	-	4
Total	39	6	45

As it is evident by the Table - 1 the maximum patients 14 were in age group of 21 to 30 years range followed by the patients of 4th decade of their life.

3. TYPE OF FISTULA :

As per the Ayurvedic description the varities of fistulae studied were all but Shataponaka. There were 14 No. of Usthagreeva or Pittaja fistulae, and 25 No. of Parisravee or kaphaja type of fistulae. There were two shanbugavartaka type and 4 unmargi type. (Table 2).

As per the anotomical situation of fistulae is concerned there were 8 subcutuneous or submucus, 14 Lowanal and 13 high and fistulae. There were 10 ano rectal fistulae (Table 3).

Table : 2 Type of fistulae :

No.	Type	Male	Female	Total
1.	Ushtragreeve (Pittajs)	12	2	14
2.	Pasisravi (Khaphaja)	22	3	25
3.	Shanbuka avartaka (Tridoshaj)	2	-	02

4.	Unmargi (Kshataja)	3	1	04
	Total	39	6	45

Table : 3 Anotomical Type :

No.	Type	Male	Female	Total
1.	Sub mucus/ sub cutaneous	6	2	8
2.	Low Anal	13	1	14
3.	High Anal	11	2	13
4.	Anorectal	9	1	10
	Total	39	6	45

The highest incidence was of parisravi type and of low Anal type of fistuale.

4. CHRONICITY OF FISTULAE.

Among the cases studied for the present tiral maximum chronic was a male case who was bering the tract for 10 years, but rest of the cases mostly were having the history of fistula around 3 to 5 years. There were also cases who got the Ischeorectal, perinanl abcesses drained and formal fistula. They were grouped under the chronicity from 0-2 years. (Table 4).

Table : 4. Cronicity of the patients in years :

No.	Chronicity	Male	Female	Total
1.	0-2 yrs	12	3	15
2.	2-3 yrs	8	1	9
3.	3-4 yrs	6	1	7
4.	4-5 yrs	12	-	12
5.	5yrs and above	1	1	2
Total		39	6	45

Recurrence before Kshara sutra treatment :

Out of 45 patients 28 patients got their problem for atleast second time. Out of this 20 have had surgery at various centres but again had it back. 8 were taking Palliative treatment. In about 3 patients the surgery was conducted 3 times or more. (Table - 5)

Table : 5 Previous Recurrence

No.	Recurrence	Male	Female	Total
1.	Operation Once or twice	14	1	15
	Palliative treatment	6	2	8
2.	Operation Thrice or more	4	1	5
	Palliative] treatment	-	-	-
	Total	24	4	28

6. pH values :

The pH values of all the ingrediants used in preparation of the applicant of the thread was estimated before the smearing. The pH value of individual ingrediants and the mixture is measured separately. For all the batches of thread prepared for this study. (Table-6)

Table - 6 pH values of Kshara Sutra ingrediants

No.	Name	pH value
1.	Haridra (Turmeric Powder Added to water)	6.2
2.	Latex expressed from Tendre Papaya fruit	6.8
3.	Tankan Kshara dissolved in water	7.4
4.	Total mixture of all the above	7.3

Thus the prepared Kshara Sutra's pH value was nearly 7.3. (Alkaline)

7. Unit cutting Time :

A) Length of fistulae : The fistulae were of various lengths ranging 3.5 cm to 16 cm. The anorectal fistulae were above 10 cm.

B) UCT : The UCT is estimated by deviding the total number of days (average) in each anotomical group by the average length of the fistula in that group. Therefore the average UCT of each group is estimated. For submucus/ subcuterneous type, the UCT is 2.97 for low anal type it is 5.02, for highanal type it is 4.57 and for Anorectal verity it is 3.51 in days.

Thus the UCT was minimum in subcutuneous verity and also in anorectal variety Probably due to the fact that the tissue that is subjected for cutting there was very much lose and also due to the fact that as the length increases the total pressure on the tissue held by Kshara Sutra will be increased and thereby the cutting rate.(Table 7).

Table 7

Type		Average initial length (cms)	Average total no. of days of treatment	Average UCT	No. of cases	Percentage
1.	Submucus/ subcutunuous	4.2cm	12.75	2.97	8	7.77%
2.	Low anal	5.6cm	28.14	5.02	14	31.11%
3..	High anal	6.1cm	27.90	4.57	13	28.88%
4.	Anorectal	9.1cm	31.95	3.51	10	22.22%

Total 16.07

Average UCT : 4.0175

Thus the average UCT of the total group of patients is 4.0175 days.

8. Pains : In this study it is found that the pain felt by patients was very much low. The patients use to feel during pain soon after the change of thread for one hour later the pain was bearable. It was also noted that patient was ambulatory throughout the treatment. But however few patients were asked to stay in the hospital for 2 days at time of 1st application.

Thus the two major advantages of the Kshara Sutra treatment in fistula in ano were found to be consistant in this study also.

9. Follow up : The patients were regularly followed up for a period of 2 years starting from the 1st application of. thread, as per the schedule mentioned earlier.

Out of all the male patients 2 patients complained pain and oozing of the wound near the area. They were checked for having the tract again. But there was not tract found and the cut wound of the Kshara Sutra was active and slightly inflammed. This was treated as per the situation and got healed. All the female cases didn't complained any problem and operated area was healthy.

10. Structure or incontinence : This was not found in any of the case. The defection was normal.

SUMMARY AND CONCLUSIONS :

The following observations could be made during the study of the Kshara Sutra made by latex of Papaya.

1. The treatment was ambulatory and there was no major discomfort to the patient.

2. The amount of pain felt by the patients was minimum and there was no feeling of discomfort.

3. The pH value of latex is below 7 and the combined value of the mixture was above 7. Therefore the thread was alkaline with less burning sensation.

4. The unit cutting time (UCT) was shorter than other

threads probably due to the proteins digestive capacity of the papaya latex.

5. Two cases were with tract around the anus with single opening. Simulating with the discriptions of 'Shambukavarta' type of fistula.

6. The recurrence rate was less than 5% where complete recurrence was not observed.

7. The complications like haemorrhage, stricture and incontinence was not encountered in any case.

ACKNOWLEDGEMENT :

I am thankful to Dr. S. P. Dixit, Principal of S. V Ayurvedic Medical college, Tirupati, for his support and also to Dr. Bulusu Sitaram for his co-operation in compilation of the Drug review.

REFERENCES :

1. Despande P. J. Sharma K. R. 'Management of Fistula in one with Kshara Sutra and its different types, ayu-Jan. 1978. Oct. 1977, July 77, April 77.

2. Kulwant Singh, Jain T. C., Kshirasagar T. D., 'A Clinical study of the various methods in treatment of Bhagandara, (Fistula is ano)' AYU- July 1988, p. 13-35.

3. Tyagi N. K., Varshaney S. C. Fistula in ano management by Kshara Sutra' Journal of NIMA May 1991, Page 7-9.

4. ICMR Collaborating Centres, Central Biostatistical monitoring unit Madras. "Multicentric randomizeal clinical trial of Kshara Sutra, (Ayurvedic Medicated thread) in the management of fistula in ano." Indian journal of Medical research, (B) 94, June 91 P. P. 177-185.

5. Rochke, and Kravse H, 'Thread drainage of perianal fistula' successful ambulatory treatment of chronic disease." Asn r. t. Allegerment Medicine. Dr. Landariz. VOLXIB 384-389, 20th Oct. 1989.

[Reference : *Proceedings - 1st International Seminar on Complimentary Medicines 1995*]

Chapter : 19

Surgical Conditions

—Dr. S. R. JOSHI

रूद्ध - partial obstruction

आमपक्वाशय अन्तेषु बस्तौच सुषीरा खालू।। सु शा ५/३२

सन्निरुद्ध मुदजठर ग्रंथी क्षत दृष्यन्ते ।। सु सू २३/८

निरुणद्धि महास्त्रोत सूक्ष्मव्दारं करोतिच।

मार्गस्य सौक्ष्म्यात् संन्निरुद्ध।। सु नि १३/५५ चचि ५/६

बस्तिसंधौ रुगणाध्मानं वधति पा यते पिच। च चि १३/१८

meaning that stenosis of sphincters Situated at the end of stomach rectum or bladder results in narrowing of openings and passages and produces stretching pain and distension.

बद्ध complete obstruction

पक्ष्मबाले सहान्नेन मुक्तैः बद्धायते गुदे।।

स्त्रोतसांदूषणात् संक्षोभात् आन्त्रसंमूर्च्छनेनवा।। चचि

आन्त्र संमूर्च्छनम् इति आन्त्र परिवर्तनम्।। $\frac{13}{13-39}$

[परिवर्तनम - स चापि बाहयाभयंत भेदेन विदधा]

meaning Eating Pika, internal and external obstructive diseases of intestines or acute folding of intestines produce intestinal obstruction. The acute folding may be either intussusception or a valvulus.

बद्ध Signs and symptoms

विड्वातसंग। हृन्नाभिमध्ये परिवृद्धिमेति। सु नि ७/१८
नाभेस्मरिसप्रायः गोपुच्छाकृति जायते। असंनि
विटसमगंधिकंच प्रच्र्छदयन् बद्ध गुदी। ३२//३३
गुल्माकृति व्यंजित लक्षणानि उदराणि ।। सु नि ७/५
स्पर्शोपलभ्यः परिपिंडितत्वात् गुल्मो नाम। चचि ५/७

Obstinate constipation, abd. distension, step ladder pattern of obstructed loops, persistant vomiting e faecal smell, and a palpable mass in intussusception.

विद्रधी - Abscess

अन्तशरीरे मांसासृक प्रविशन्ति यदामलाः।
वातिकिपैत्तिकी तृष्णा दाह मोह मद ज्वरेः। च सू
अभ्यंतरेचमहच्छूलं विद्रधीषूपजायते।। $\frac{17}{93-97}$

आध्यामातं बधदनिषयंदं छर्दिहिक्कातूडान्वितम्।
रूजाश्वास समाविष्टं विद्रधीर्नाशयेत नरम।। सु सू ३३/२२

Severe pain, fever thirst and delirium are signs of internal abscess and Distension Oliguria, Vomitting Hiccough and dyspnea are serious signs [वृक्क उडुक & क्लोक विद्रधी]

Site of Pain

हृदये क्लोम्नि यकृति प्लीही वृक्कौच कुक्षयोः च सू
नाभ्यां वंक्षणयोर्वा पि बस्तौवा तीव्र वेदना १७/९४

हृदयेक्लोम्नि is pain in epigastric region, यकृति प्लीही is Rt or Lt hypochondriac region, कुक्षौ is Rt or Lt parqcolic region वृक्कौ is in the region of kidneys नाभ्यां is umbilical वंक्षणयो : is Rt or Lt iliac region बस्तौ is suprapublic region.

Thus the regional distribution of pain is related to the underlying etiopathology.

Etiopathology

Underlying etiopathological causes may be

ब्रभछिद्र रुद्धबद्ध विध्र विद्ध गुल्म ग्रंथस्तिथा।

कृमि ब्रध्नाश्म विट् आम भ्रंशसंग अगंतवा।।

व्रणछिद्र (Ulcer and perforation) रुद्धबद्ध (Partialor complete obstruction) विध्रविद्ध (Abscess and stab injury) गुल्मग्रंथी (Globular or cystic swelling) कृमी (Worms) ब्रध्नअश्मरी (Strangulation and calculus) विट्आम (Hyperperistaltic) भ्रंशसंग (Ectopic gestation) आगंतू (External / Accidental)

व्रण - Ulcer

अभोजनादजीर्णातिभोजनात् व्दिष माशनात्। चचि १५/४४

अपच्यमानं शुक्तत्वं याति अन्नं विषकपतास्।

विषदिध्देन पच्यते [आन्त्रं] गत्वा मांसंच कृष्णताम। असंउ ४०/१०७

आरक्त पीत पर्यतः श्याबमध्ये अतिरूक व्रणः।।

भुक्तमात्रे अथवा वान्ते जीर्णेन्नेवा प्रशाम्यति। मानिशूल

Irregularity in eating habbits causes hyperacidity and pain. Ulcer is caused by mucosal digestion of stomach or duod by extremely acidic and acrid nature of Pitta e severe pain.

छिद्र - विद्ध perforation, puncture.

अस्थादिशल्यै सान्नैश्च भुक्ते अत्यशनेनवा। असंनि १२/३४

भिद्यते पच्यते चान्त्रं तद्र छिद्रैश्च स्त्रवत्‌बहिः।

इयात् [अन्न] पाकं रसस्तेभ्यः छिद्रेभ्यः प्रस्त्रवेत् बहिः।

रसो आन्त्रपाकं उदरान्तरे प्रसृतं उदरं जनयति। चचि १३/४३

आहार मूत्र पुरीष दर्शनमूच व्रणमुख्यात्। सु सू २६/१०

perforation is caused by eating pika or by rupture of an ulcer or an abscess and the intestinal contents leak into abd. cavity puncture may be by stab or bull gore injury

पित्ताश्मरी - गोरोचनेव

रोचनेव गवांपित्ते ...... अश्मर्य संभवन्त्यथा का चि पत्र १२१

कुक्षौ हृन्नाभिमध्येषु स शूल कपमैत्किः मा नि शूल

दौर्बल्य अल्पाग्नि पार्श्वार्ति हिध्माश्वासरुचिज्वरै।

तिलपिष्ट निभंयस्तु कामलावान् सृजेत मलम।। वा चि १६/४५-४७

Colicky pain of Biliary calculus is severe in epigastric and Rt hypochondriac regions, it is also refered to Rt scapular region. When it obstructs the Biliqry passage jaundice nousia hiceough and clay coloured stools are common signs

विट्आम - कुक्षीशूल विट्शूल

यदाअस्य भोजनं भुक्तं सोपस्तंभं न पच्यते।

उच्छूसित्याम शकृता शूलेन आहन्यते मुहूः। सु उ

नैवासने न शयने तिष्ठन् वा लभते सुखाम्। $\frac{42}{124-125}$

विट्शूलं परमदारुणं शूलं तत्र सघोषवृत्।

पिपासावधति तीव्राभ्रमोमूर्च्छाच जायते। सु उ

उच्चारितो मूत्रितस्य न शांतिं अधिगच्छति। ४२/१३८-१३९

Intestinal colicky pain is due to indigestion and Hyperperistalysis. Mucus colitis and ulcerative colitis are serious diseases.

भ्रंशपरासंग - Ectopic gestation

स विमुक्तबंधनो गर्भाशयम अतिक्रम्य यकृत -
प्लीहान्त्र विवरैः अवस्त्रंसमानः कोष्ठ संक्षोभं आपादयति।
तस्या जठर संक्षोभात् वपयुः अपानो मूढः।। सु नि. ८/४

Bhransha is displacement and Parasanga is abnormal attachment. Thus extrauterine pregnancy implanted in abdominal cavity and attached to abdominal viscera causes severe pain and may obstruct the passage of food flatus and faeces.

भ्रंशपरासंग - मक्कल्ल - Ectopic rapture

गर्भकोश परासंगो मक्कल्ला योनि संवृतिः।
हन्यात् त्रियं मूढगर्भे यथोक्ताश्चाप्युपद्रवाः। सु सू ३३/१३
कोषस्य गर्भस्य स्वस्थानात् परस्थानं गत्वा
संगो इति परासंगः। कोषः पिण्डवत् विदतीये मासि। सु शा ३/१८
मक्कल्लो रक्तमास्तजशूल विशेषः।। मा नि. मूढगर्भ

Makkalla is acute abdominal pain with severe hemorrhage. Rupture of a cocoon size two month tubal pregnancy produces severe pain hemorrhage and shock

Acute Abdomen In Ayurveda

नैवासने न शयने तिष्ठने वा लभते सुखास्
तीव्र शूलोदरम सु उ ४२

He sits, He Sleeps, He stands
Tubmling the body and the hand
But Alas no relief from pain
and this is called acute Abdomen.

Ippographic Referance of Acute abdomen.

एवं प्रकुपिताः तांस्तान् शरीर प्रदेशान् आगम्य
तांस्तान् व्याधीन् जनयन्ति। ते यदा उदर
सन्निवेशं कुर्वन्ति तदा गुल्म विद्रधी उदरशूल
प्रभूतीन् जनयन्ति तं वक्षामः।। सु सू २१/२३

Meaning that the Pathogens have some specific affinity to-wards some organs in Human body - when they find their way in Abdomen they cause Gulma, Vidhradhi shoola etc. Tossing and excruciating pain in abdomen is Acute abdomen. In Ayurveda it is known as Mahat shoolam, Maharuja or Teevra Vedana and is naturally related to the Intrabodminal structures. In Ayurveda the Intraabodominal organs are

यकृतप्लीहोंदुक वृक्कौ नाभि [क्लामे] डिभांत्र बस्तयः। वा शा ३/१२

स्त्रीणाम् आवृत्यतिष्ठंति फलं अंतर्गतं हि ता। सु शा ५/४१

liver, spleen, caecum, kidneys, pancrea, pelvic colon Intestines Bladder ovaries and Fallopian tubes.

Type of Pain.

शंक्वास्फेटनवत्तस्य यस्मात् तीव्राश्च वेदनाः।

वायुप्रकुपितो कोष्ठे शूलं संजनयेत् भृशस्। सु उ

निरुच्छ्वासो भवेत तेन वेदना पिडीतो नरः। ४२/८०-८१

क्रुप्दो वायु कर्तनायामतोदैः

कम्पाध्म्रानैराविशन् कुक्षिदेशे। का. खिल २८/४

मक्कल्लो रक्तमासतज शूल विशेषः। मा. नि. मूढगर्भ

Acute abdominal pain may be bursting cutting stretching throbing or colicky and is usually accompained by Breath Holding and tremors

गुल्मग्रंथी - lump in Abd.

गुल्मे अन्तराश्रये बस्तिकुक्षीहृदप्लीह वेदना। असंनि. ११/४३

अग्नि वर्ण बलींश वेगानाच अप्रवर्तनस्।।

श्वासशूल पिपासान्न विव्देष ग्रंथी मूढता:। सु सू ३३/२१
भवन्ति दुर्बलत्वंच गुल्मिनो मृत्यु मेष्यत:

An intraabdominal tumor, growth or a globular mass may produce pain in different regions and obstruct intestinal or urinary passage. A fixed tumor with pain, dyspnea, thirst and anoxaxia is dangerous

कृभि - Worms

ज्वरो विवर्णता शूलं हृद्रोगं सदनं भ्रम:।
भक्तव्देषो अतिसादश्च संजात कृमिलक्षणम। सु उ ५४/१८
आन्यादा उदरावेष्टा हृदयादा महाकुहा।
विड्भेदशूल विष्टभ कार्म्य पारुष्य पांडुता। वानि
रोमहर्षोग्निसदन गुद कंडू विनिर्गमात्। $\frac{14}{49-56}$

Acute abd pain is common with round worm infestation of intestines. Anemia and perianal itch are also common and fever diarrhea or constipation may be present

ब्रध्न - Obstructed hernia.

ब्रध्नो अनिलाघौ: वृषणे स्वलिंगै: आन्त्रंनिरेति। च चि १२/९४
मूत्रेणपूर्ण मृदू मेदसा तू स्निग्धं विद्यात् कठिनंच शोथं।
आन्त्रवृद्धिदरसाध्यो यं वातबृष्टि समाकृति:
रुक्षकृष्पारुग्णसिरातन्तु जाल गवाक्षित:। अ. सं नि ११/३३

Bradhna means obstructed scrotal hernia
It is either enterocele cystocele or Omentocele
A tense tender and painful hernia is strangulated hernia. In gangrene it become congested Blue and Black and a gangrene Perforation is incurable

मूत्रश्मरी - मूत्रशूल - बस्तिशूल

नाभ्यां वंक्षण पार्श्वेषु कुक्षौ भेद्रान्त्रमर्दकः।

मूत्र आवृत्त गृहणाति मूत्रशूल स मारुतात। सु उ $\frac{42}{134-135}$

बस्ति वंक्षण नाभिषु ततः शूलो अस्य जायते।

विण्मूत्र वात संरोधि बस्तिशूल स मारुतात्।

प्रसूनानाभिवृषणं रुद्धमूत्रं अश्यरी सरुम्।। सु सू ३३/१२

pain due to calculus in urinary tract is Renal colic Back pain, Loin to groin pain and pain in tip of penis are the typical signs of calculu situated at different levels,

आगंतुकं - External & accidental

आगंतुकं [आघातेन छिन्नभिन्नादि] सप्तमं उदरं। सु नि ७/४

रूणद्धि मारुतश्लेष्मा कुक्षिपार्श्व व्यवस्थितः। सु उ ४२/१७

सुचिभिरिव निस्तोदं कृछ्रोश्वासी तदा नर] पार्श्वशूल

हृदयस्तु संघातं परिक्षीणस्य देहिनाम्। भे इं ४/९

अत्यर्थ पीडयेत् शूलं सद्यः प्राणान् जहितिसः। हृदशूल

Finally the acute abdomen may be due to accidental injury to abdominal viscera or it may be a refered pain from chest eg. Diaphragmatic pleurisy or Angina Pectoris.

[Reference : International Seminar 1995]

Chapter : 20

Marma Vidnyan

Dr. V. V. Doiphode

Marma Vidnyan is the peculiarity of Ayurveda. In so other medical science, this aspect is structed. This subject deals with particular sites in the body, which are to be avoided while performing surgical procedures. The knowledge of Anatomy is required for diagnosing different diseases, as well as for surgery. The topic is discussed by Sushruta in sharir sthan, some references are also available in Charak Samhita and Ashtang hridaya.

In ancient literatures including Veda & Buddhist works, various reference regarding Anatomy are found. Quotations of descriptive Anatomy have been found in commentaries written over thousand years ago on surgical works like Bhela Samhita - Dr. Hoernley in his book 'Medicine in ancient India' quotes 'probably it will come as a surprise to many, as, it did to myself, to discover the amount of anatomical knowledge which is so descriptive and correct in ancient Indian literature.

The word Marma is derived from the sanskrit root 'Mru' means to kill - 'Marayanti Iti Marmani.' It is applied to a place of vital importance in the body, which, if injured results in serious consequences, or death, sooner or later.

JEEVANASTHANAM TU MARMASYAT

- Rajnighantu

Sushrut defines 'marma' as a place where mamsa, sira, snayu, asthi, sandhi are present. They are the seats of concentration of Pranic currents and Bhootatma, (Supreme power or force controlling the body and mind). Therefore injury to marma results in death.

Marma is a vital point or place in the body which when hurt ultimately kills the person. The results of injury very from severe pain to sudden death. This result of injury or blow is because these places are the sites, where fleshy parts, certain sira, snayu, bones and joints are intermingled with one another.

Naturally, the important organs or groups of important structures rae held together hence if they receive a blos, or an injury they will cause serious ill-effects on the body. The symptoms produced by injury to a marma are peculiar to the place where marma is situated. All marmas are more or less the seats of 'Prana', that means they are in close association with chetana, due to this fact, injury to marma produces severe sufferings.

Considering the origin and practical utility of marmas, charaka gives great importance to these marmas namely Basti (Bladder), Hridaya (Heart), Shira (Head) and they are included in the Ten Pranayatan (Seats of life). He considered them of Paramount importance from treatment point of view in as much as the vitiated doshas affect the marma and cause diseases which may prove fatal.

Surgically it is of more practical use. An injury to any marma may result in death immediately or later by complications or end in deformity of a particular part of the body. Injuries of equally severe nature else where in the body, need not necessarilyy prove fatal provided marma in these parts are in-tact. Surgeons of ancient India led down the rule, that in case of a surgical operation, the situation and dimension of each local marma should first be studied well and the incision for operation should be made in such a way as to avoid even the age of a marma.'

The knowledge of marma was practically made use of in ancient warfare and in hunting after wild animals, by hitting the enemy aiming at the marma. This science is also practised in the art of wrestling (Ji-Jutsu).

The panchabhautic classification of marma is, that, it contains the elements of Prithvi, Apa, Teja and Vaju, predominantly. It also contains Triguna i.e. Satwa, Raja and Tama and they are the seats of Atma. Hence person does not live when the marma are hurt.

All the marmas are included in Madhyama-Vyadhi-marg along with heart, bladder, joints etc. Diseases in the Madhyama Marga are difficult for treatment. There are three Vyadhi Marga - Bahya, Abhyantara and Madhyama. Prognosis of the diseases or ease of treatment is directly proportional to the Marga.

The diseases or injuries to the organs of which marma is composed are difficult to treat and many a times are not curable.

NUMBER OF MARMAS

Total number of marmas in the body is 107 and they are distributed in the body as follows :

A. Each Extremity 11	44
B. Abdomen & Thorax	12
C. Back	14
D. Head & Neck	37
	107

CLASSIFICATION OF MARMA

The marmas are classified mainly according to the structure by which they are formed and by the effect of the blow.

Human body is composed mainly by saptadhatu and is controlled by the functions of Tridosha. There are other body building tissues also. Almost every tissue in the body is part and parcel of saptadhatu either in the form of upadhatu or Mala and hence every structure has to be made out of Saptadhatu.

Tridosha control the functions in body and hence they also have direct action on tissue formation.

Marmas classified according, to the structures they are formed of, is as follows :

Mansa Marma	11
Sira Marma	41
Asthi Marma	08
Snayu Marma	27
Sandhi Marma	20
	107

Thus sira marma contains sira (i.e. vessels) predominantly in its structure, hence when injury occurs the resultant rupture of the vessel causes blood loss or spillage of the fluid contents in the vessel. This loss of important fluids in the body will result in other complications.

Injury to anayu marma will lead to muscle tear or deformities in muscles which will lead to paralysis.

Injuries to Asthi or Sandhi will lead to fractures and/ or dislocations leading to deformities, severe pain, and in case of shock, death sooner or later.

Besides these, there are no other structural varieties according to Subhruta. According to Vagbhata, there is one more variety which he calls as 'Dhamani marma'.

The marmas are also classified according to the results they cause after an injury or a blow. They are of 5 types.

(1) SADDYA PRANAHARA

Which causes immediate death. According to Sushruta there are 19 in number.

(2) KALANTARA PRANAHARA

In the variety, the resultant death occurs after some times. They are in all 33 in numbers as per Sushruta Samhita.

(3) WISHALL YAGHNA

In this variety symptoms are not experienced as long as the foreign body which has made a blow on the body is at the site. Death or serious results occur as soon as the foreign body is removed. The object seals the wound itself, preventing important fluids present in the object to come out. Attempt of forceful removal of the foreign body causes symptoms due to spillage of internal fluids.

According to Sushruta, they are 3 in number.

(4) VAIKALL YAKARA

Effect of blow on this marma results in permanent loss of a limb or its activity. As per Sushruta Samhita they are 44 in number.

(5) RUJAKARA

The blow results in severe pain - They are in all 8 according to Sushruta.

Saddya Pranahara marma after an injury causes death immediately or within a week. In case of Kalantara Pranahara marma death occurs within 2-4 weeks. In this variety time of the resultant death will depend upon the severity of blow. A severe blow will cause sudden death in this variety also.

Though Vishallyaghna and Vaikallyakara marmas do not cause fatal results, if the injury is severe, they may also lead to resultant death. The symptoms or results after a blow on marma vary according to the situation of the injury in the marma. If the marma is injured at the periphery, the results are not that severe, e.g. an injury at the periphery of the Saddya pranahara marma will not cause sudden death. It may give rise to symptoms of blow on a Kalantara pranahara marma. Similarly injury at Kalantara pranahara marmas will cause symptoms of a blow on Vaikalyakara marma. A blow at the periphery of Vaikalyakara marma will produce symptoms that are produced after a blow on Rujakara marma. If the blow is at the centre of the marma, the resultant symptoms will be according to the name of the marma.

In Saddya pranahara marma, the principal Mahabhoot is Agni, Due to quick disappearance of Agni qualities, instant death occurs after a blow. In Kalaṇtara pranahara marma, there is predominence of Agni and Soma. Though Agni quality disappears quickly, some quality persists for some time to prolong the life. The Wishalyaghna marma does not cause fatal effects as long as the foreign body remains in situ. Its presence seals the opening of the cavity (Ashaya) which does not cause serious effects. The moment the foreign body is removed, it gives an opening in that cavity. Vayu in that cavity escapes through the opening resulting into Ashayariktata, which causes fatal effects. In Vaikalyakara marmas there is a predominence of soma quality, the loss this quality causes loss of injured limb only. Soma being naturally cold and rigid closes the opening and does not allow Atma to pass away and hence in there varieties severe blows also do not cause death.

In Rujakara variety Agni and Vayu are in predominence and hence they cause severe pain. According to some scientists this pain is due to the presence of All Pancha mahabhutas.

Sushruta has given the sites of different marmas elaborately. The marmas are situated throughout the body.

He has explained the sites of particular marma and its extent with the help particular marma and its extent with the help of Anguli pramana. An Anguli means transverse distance at the middle of index finger of the examiner. This information is as per Charak, Vagbhata differs from this measurement, according to him an Anguli is the transverse distance of the ring finger. According to Sushruta, it is the little finger which is made use of to denote the Anguli pramana.

Though the result of the blow are explained as sudden death, late death etc. We do not observe these results routinely. It seems that the results vary according to the severity of the blow also. Even on the Saddya pranahara marma, if the blow is not more severe, it may not give rise to sudden death as we observe in day to day life. Heart is a Saddya pranahara marma. A blow on the chest wall at the position of Heart should cause sudden death, this fact is not rountinely observed, instead, a minor blow does not cause any effect whatsoever, still the heart is regarded as a site, where after an injury death is certain. In case of accidental stoppage of heart (Heart block) a gentle massage (blows of less severity) on the chest wall behind which heart is situated causes stimulation of cardiac musculature and thereby refunctioning of the circulatory system. Thus a gentle blow on a Saddya pranahara marma instead of causing ill effects helps to stimulate the stopped functions of an important organ to prevent death. This proves that the sites of marma are improtant not only from surgical point of view but also have therapeutic importance. Gentle blows will act as massage on these organs thereby stimulating the stopped functions; a useful fact for treatment in averting different diseases of the body. In this respect the knowledge of marma is comparable to accupuncture therapy. In case of accupressure therapy, marma vidnyan is important. A pressure exerted at a particular marma will relieve pain and other symptoms of the organ concerned.

The marma are explained in different parts of the body.

Each limb (extremity) there are 11 marmas (In all 44 in 4 limbs). Their names are Kshipra; Talahridaya, Koorch; Koorchashira; Gulf; Indrabasti; Janu; Aani; Urvi; Rohitaksha; Vitapa (in lower limb).

There is a peculiar method to explain the marma, for example - Kshipra marma is explained as follows :

(A) STHAN (SITE; PLACE)

Between nedex finger and thumb.

(B) PRAKARA (TYPE)

1. According to effect - Kalantara Pranahara
2. According to tissue - Snayu.

(C) PRAMANA (EXTENT)

Ardhanguli - about 1 cm

(D) PRAINAMA (EFFECTS)

Injury leads to cionic spasms of sup. ext. and late death.

In case of superior extremity the names of few marmas are different than those in inf. ext. such as Manibandha (Gulfa); Koorpar (Janu); Bavhi (Urvi); Kakshadhara (Vitapa).

In this manner every marma is – explained.

There are 12 marmas in abdomen and Thorax; they are - Guda; Basti; Nabhi; Hridaya and Stanamoola; Stanarohita; Apalap and Apasthambha in duplicate.

Marmas in the back are 14 (they are in pairs. Their names are Katikataruna; Kukundara; Nitamba; Parshwasandhi; Brihati; Amsa-phalaka and Amsa.

Marmas in head and neck means the marmas situated above clavicle are :

Dhamani (4 in number) Matruka (8 in number)
Krikatika (2 in number) Vidhura (2 in number)
Phana (2 in number) Apanga (2 in number)
Avarta (2 in number) Utkkshepa (2 in number)
Shankha (2 in number) Sthapani (2 in number)
Seemanta (5 in number) Shringataka (4 in number)
Adhipati (1 in number)

Every marma is explained as per the explanation given about the Kshipra marma.

A comparison of marma explanation and anatomical structure - will be useful to know exact information. For this comparison vitapa marma will be useful.

According to sushruta the vitapa marma is explained as follows :

Sthana (Site)

Between Vankshna & Vrishana (Between groin and acrotum)

Prakara -

i. Snayu (Vagbhata calls it as sira marma)

ii. Vaikalyakara

Parimana (Extent) -

1. Anguli (About 2 cm)

Parinama (Effect) -

Ruja (Pain); Alpashukrata (Oligosperimoea) or Shandhya (Impotency)

The situation of this marma is between Tastes (Scrotum) & groin. Injury to this marma leads to impotency (moderate or severe) and pain. Anatomical structures corresponding to this marma-

1. Fasciase binding the several structures of the spermatic cord namely -
    a. intercrural fascia
    b. cremasteric fascia
    c. infundibuliform fascia
2. Testicular artery and vein.
3. The ductus difference and the artery supplying it.
4. Testecular nerve.

Considering the structures around the marma injury of these structures will cause stoppage of the flow of sperms from tastes to urethra. This in turn will lead to impotency. Injury to the nerve will cause pain, severe or moderate. Cutting of Vas-defference accidentally or deliberately will cause obstruction to the flow of sperms. In case of females, this is the site of round ligament. It is because of this ligament that the position of Anteversion of uterus is maintained. Cutting of this ligament will cause retroversion. Persistent retroversion is definite cause of sterility in females. In case of primipara during delivery, trausmatic injury to this marma can occur, this injury is called as Vitapabheda. In this case sever pain and subsequent sterility results. To avoid this complication of vaginal tear an operation is performed in which a cut is resulted in vaginal wall which increases the passage for foetus avoiding transmatic rupture of the vitapa marma. This operation is called an Episiotomy.

Unfortunately this comparison is not posible for most of the marmas. In this advanced era of sophisticated operations, the danger of marmaghata is reduced. Even amputation of a limb does not cause death. Even today precautions before taking an incision are explained, incision should avoid the marma area is an accepted fact.

In case of stapani marma, which is a Wishalyaghna

marma. Situated around frontal air sinus. Trauma due to Foreign body will cause marmaghat, forceful attempt of removal of the F. B. will take out the contents alongwith Prana and thereby cause death. In day to day practice, we observe that the sinuses are washed during sinuritis which relieves the pain, if the contents are taken out to relieve symptoms how marmaghat will occur? In this case the knowledge of marma helped to cure the disease.

It is also difficult to locate the exact marma organ, whether it is frontal air sinus, meninges, frontal lobe or the brain substance behind that is not clearly known.

In today's life we definitely can use the marma knowledge during surgery to protect important organs as well as in therapeutics for stimulating the functions of the organ by applying gentle blow; a treatment comparable to accupressure.

[Reference : Deerghayu International Vol. 8/2, April-June 1992]

Chapter : 21

Introduction to Shalakya Tantra

–Dr. D. P. Puranik

This is one of the eight branches of Ashtang Ayurved.

The name Shalakya is derived from the word "Shalaka" which means a rod like structure and so, the branch of Ayurvedic science is called as 'Shalakya-tantra' since us of 'Shalaka' is predominant in treatment.

'Shalakya-Tantra' comprises study of diseases of those parts of body which occur above suprasternal notch i.e. Urdhvajatrugat vyadhi. So, this branch consists study of the diseases of 'Mukh' (Throat), Nasa (Nose), Karna (Ear), Netra (Eye) and Shir (Head). Since all these organs are of prime importance it is also called as 'Uttamang Chikitsa'.

Shalakya-Tantra is also popularly known as 'NIMITANTRA' since king NIMI is supposed to be the pioneer and great authority on Shalakya-Tantra.

Videh is also an authority and so the science is also called as 'Videh-tantra'.

Sushrutacharya - famous surgeon, Charakacharya, Vagbhatacharya have also elaborated the subject to great extent.

Other ancient authorities on Shalakya-Tantra include Karal, Bhadrak, Shaunak, Bhoj etc.

The person who treats is called as Shalaki.

Nose is supposed to be the main outlet (Dwar) for head region (Nasa hi Shirasa Dwaram) and so it becomes main source for the administration of the drugs in the treatment of ear, nose, throat, eyes and head.

After the introduction to the subject we proceed to know salient features of all the parts individually and separately.

Mukh-Roga (Diseases of Throat)

According to Ayurvedic anatomy Mukh comprises oshtha (Lips), Dantamoola (Alveolar process and gums), Danta (Teeth), Tongue (Jivha), Taloo (Palate), Kanth (Laryngeal part) and remaining Mukh.

Common etiological factors (Hetoo) - Excessive consumption of alcohols, pork, fish, curds, milk, sugarcaine juice, bad oral hygiene etc.

General symptoms and signs (Samanya laxane) -

Excessive salivation, reluctance to breast feeding or food, expulsion of milk from nose or vomitting etc.

Oshtha Rogas (Diseases of Lips) - These are Oshthakopa, - Different types, Khandaushtha (Hare-Lip), Arbuda (Tumour), Jalarbud (Cyst) etc.

Principles of treatment -

Raktamoksha (Blood letting)

Snehan, Swedan, Lep (application of paste)

Dantamoolgata Rogas (Affections of gums and Alveolar process) :- Old granthas mention 15 different diseases. These include sheetad (Bleeding gums), Dantapupput (Gum Boil), Danta Veshtak (Pyorrhoea Alveolaris), Vardhan (Extra tooth), Adhimansak (Impacted wisdom), Dantavidradhi (Alveolar abscess), Danta-nadi (sinus) etc.

Treatment in general - Raktamoksha (Blood letting) is principle treatment Gandush and Kaval (Gargles and holding medicinal solution in mouth).

Pratisaran (Application of paste or dusting).

Nasya (Nasal drops).

Dantagat Roga (Diseases of teeth) - These rogas include Dalan (Toothache), Krimidant (caries tooth), Dantaharsh (Odontitis), Bhanjanak, Dantasharkara (Tartar), Kapalika (Enamel separation), Shyavdant, Hanumoksha (Dislocation of mandible).

Simple and Common Treatment - Vatanashak treatment, Kavalgrahan (Holding medicated oil or solution in mouth).

Diseases to Tongue (Jivha Roga) - These include Jivha Kantak - 3 (Superficial glossitis), Alas (sublingual abscess), Upjivha (Ranula or Salivary cyst), Adhijivha.

Treatment - Principal treatment is Raktamoksha by lekhan karma (Blood letting).

Kaval & Gandush (Gargles & holding solution in mouth).

Pratisaran (Application of medicine)

Nasya (Nasal drops)

Talu Rogas (Diseases of palate) - Total 8 diseases are described. These include Galashundika (Elongated Uvula), Tundikeri (Enlarged tonsils), Adrush, Kaschap (Sarcoma), Arbud (Cancer), Mansanghat (Adenoma of palate), Talupupput (Epulis of palate), Talushosh, Talupak (Ulceration), Talupitika, Talushoth.

Treatment - Nasya, Gandush, Lekhan (scrapping), Chhedan (Excision of diseased part), Avapidan.

Kanthagat Rogas (Diseases of Larynx) - Sushrutacharya has described 17 rogas. These include Rohini (Diphtheria), Kanthashaluk (Enlarged adenoids), Valay, Balas, Ekvrund, Vrund, Shataghni, Gilayu (Acute Tonsillitis). Galavidradhi (Phyaryngeal abscess), Galaugh, Swaraghna, Mook-minmin, gadgad, Manstan, Vidari, Galarbud (Tumour), Galagraha (Pharyngitis).

General treatment -

Raktamoksha (Blood letting).

Nasya.

Kaval, Pratisaran.

Orally Kwath.

Sarvasar (Stomatitis) -

Vataj Sarvasar - Ulcerative stomatitis

Pittaj Sarvasar - Gangrenous stomatitis

Kaphaj - Apthous Ulcer.

Treatment - Cleaning of mouth i.e. mouth wash.

Kaval - Gandush.

Pratisaran.

Internally - Kamdudha Kalp, Khadiradi Guti.

Nasa Roga (Diseases of Nose) - These diseases include Pratishyay (Acute Rhinitis), Apeenas, Pootinasya (ozaena), Nasapak, Raktapitta, Pooyrakta, Kshavathu, Deept, Nasarsh (Nasal polyp), Nasarbud (New growths).

Etiological Factors i.e. Hetoo - Extremely cold climate, Dusty and foggy surroundings, Loud Speech, Day time sleep, change in habits, Low resistance and immunity, Allergy, Chr. diseases etc.

Treatment - Snehan, Swedan (Steam inhalation), Abhyang, Diet - Wheat-Rice, Light, warm diet containing, - Ghee and Salt.

Apathya-To Avoid - Pitta dosha stimulant & drying of local Kapha. Consumption of alcohols, coffee, Tea, Tobacco, Banana, Potato, Ice cold water, Dipping in cold water.,

Karna Roga (Diseases of ear) - Total 15 different rogas are described and 5 rogas that of Karnapali i.e. pinna of ear. These include - karnashool (pain in ear),

Pranad or Karna nad (Tinitus), Karnabadhirya (Deafness), karnkshwed (Labrynthitis), Karnastrav (Otorrhoea), Kărnakandoo (Itching), Karna varchas, Krimikarna (Maggots in ear), Pratinah (Eustachian tube obstruction), Vidradhi (Furuncle), Karna pak (Suppuration), Pootikarna (Foetid discharge), Karnarsh (Ear polyp), Karnarbud (Tumour), Karna shof.

Etiological Factors (Hetoo) - Swimming in cold water, rubbing and scratching the ear, inserting sticks or rods in ear, exposure to cold etc.

General treatment - Ghritpan (Consumption of Ghee), Rest, Application of oil of head, Swedan (steam), Karnapooran (Instillation of ear drops or stuffing with powder). Rechan, Vaman (vomitting), Diet -Ghee, Wheat, Rice, Chyavanprash Rasayan, Triphala etc.

Apathya-Avoid - Exercise, Rough dental cleaning, Dipping the head in cold water, Fast Wind etc.

Netra Rogas - (Diseases of eye) - As compared to Ear, Nose, Throat diseases one gets very detailed account of Netra Rogas in Sushrut Samhita. Vagbhat and Charak Samhitas also reveal very useful references in the description and treatment of ophthalmic diseases. Sushrutacharya has described 76 netra rogas.

According to Sushrutacharya Abhishyanda (Conjunctivitis) is the primary cause or predisposing factor for developing other diseases and so it is advised to treat this primary cause with utmost care to avoid further complications.

Etiological factors for eye diseases - Swimming immediately after working in bright sunlight or heat. Strainuous reading. Daytime sleep. Crying for long time. Anger, Mourning, Dust, Smoke, Withholding reflexes like micturation, defaecation, Trauma to head etc.

Primary Signs and Symptoms - Watering from eyes, Haziness in eyes, Redness in eyes, Pain, itching, burning sensation in the eye.

General treatment - Snehan, Swedan (Fomentation), Siramoksha (Blood letting).

Netrabasti (eye enemation)

Dhuma (Fumigation)

Aschotana (Instillation)

Shirobasti

Anjana (Collyrium)

Lepa (Application of paste)

Parisheka (Continuous instillation).

Alongwith medical treatment operative treatment like chhedan (Excision), Bhedan (Cutting), Lekhan (Scrapping) are also described in detail for the diseases which are not curable with medical treatment.

Shirorogas (Diseases of Head) - These include Vataj, Pittaj, Kaphaj, Sannipatik, Krimij, Raktaj, Kshayaja Shirorogas, Sooryavarta, Anantwat, Ardhavbhedak, Shankhak.

General Etiological factors - Day sleep, avoiding night sleep, excessive consumption of alcohol, loud speech, fast winds, working in extreme temperature, dusty & smoky atmosphere, Drinking ice-cold water, trauma to head, long cry, mental tension, transporation, dipping head in water.

General treatment -

Nasya (Shirovirechana) - Mustard oil

Snehan

Swedan (Fomentation)

Rakta moksha

Prevention and diet -

Advice - Swedan, Nasya, Dhoompan, Virechan,

Lepan, Parisheka, Langhan, Shirobasti, Diet - Ghee, Milk, Grapes, Mango, Buttermilk, Tail, Coconut, Sandle, Camphor.

SIMPLE REMEDIES IN SHALAKYA TANTRA -

Problems of Nose -

Pratishyay - Stuffy nose discharge etc.

(1) Vacha - (Latin Name - Acorus calamus) - Stem or powder of it, is used as a 'Nasya' - clears off nose.

(2) Tulsi - (Latin Name - Ocimum Sanctum) (English - Holy Basil.)

- Fresh juice along with honey can be given orally.
- Kwath (Decoction) of Tulsi can be given orally.
- Expressed juice can be used for 'Nasya'.
- Medicated steam can also be inhaled.

(3) Haridra (Turmeric) - (Latin Name - Curcuma Longa) - Rhizome is generally used. Roasted Haridra is given orally along with Jaggery for cough and colds (1 G. Haridra + 5G. Jaggery).

(4) Nilgiri - (Eucalyptus Rosteata) - Leaves of it are used. Extracted oil of it is used for 'Nasya' and medicated steam for inhalation - Clears choked nose due to discharge.

Epistaxis - Urdhvag Raktapitta i.e. Bleeding from nose.

(1) Durva Swaras - (Cynodon dactylon) Since it has haemostatic action, extracted juice can be used as 'Nasya'.

(2) Laksha - (Coccus Lacca) Orally - Boiled and strained.

(3) Adulsa-Vasa - (Adhatoda Vasica) - Fresh juice is used as 'Nasya'.

Allergic and Atrophic Rhinitis

- Any oil can be used as 'Nasya'.

- Sweet syrup drops also can be used.

Oropharyngeal Problems (Mukh Roga)

Pharyngitis & Tonsillitis - i.e. Galgrah & Gilayu

(1) Yashtimadhu (Glycyrrhiza Glabra) stem of it is used. Powder can be given orally along with warm water or warm milk. Stem can be used for chewing. It acts as lozenges. In case of hoarseness of voice due to Laryngitis it is given along with sugar crystals. Popular in professional singers.

(2) Haridra (Curcuma Longa) - It is given along with Jaggery or milk. It suppresses cough of pharyngeal origin. Haridra with salt is used for local application in Tonsillitis and pharyngitis. It can be used in form of 'Fant' also.

(3) Sukshma Triphala -

For Acute Tonsillitis and Pharyngitis given orally - 250 mg x 4 times daily with warm water.

(4) Cozenges - Tab. 6-8 times daily for chewing.

Dental Problem - Danta Roga

Krimi Danta and Dantashool - i.e. caries tooth & toothache.

(1) Ajmoda (Carym Copticum) - Powder is applied in cavity of caries tooth to relieve pain. Kwath (Decoction) can be given orally.

(2) Koshtha Kolinjan (Alpinia officinarum) - Rhizome of it is used. In halitosis (Bad breath) due to bad oral hygiene - Powder is applied.

Ear Problems - Karna Roga

Karna Shool (Pain in ear)

(1) Tulsi Swaras (Ocimum Sanctum) is used as ear drops to relieve pain.

(2) Lashoon (Ailiyum sativus) (Garlic) Sesame Oil + Paste can be used as Karnapooran (ear drops).

Karna Strav (Otorrhoea)

(1) Haridra (curcuma longa) - Powder is used for instillation in ear.

(2) Lashoon (Ailiyum Sativus) - Used for ear drops.

(3) Tulsi Swaras - Used as ear drops.

Shiroroga

Shirashool (Migraine)

(1) Shoonthi (Zingiber officinale) Rhizome is used.

- Extracted shoonthi juice + Onion juice + Honey to be taken orally.

- Paste i.e. Lep of Haridra + Vacha + Shoonthi can be applied on forehead.

Netra Rogas (Diseases of eye)

Netrabhishyand (Conjunctivitis)

(1) Honey - In the form of collyrium

(2) Haridrajal - Turmeric + water Boiled - Clarified Water is used in the form of eye drops.

(3) Tuwarijal - Alum + Water - Eye drops.

(4) Triphala Kwath - Decoction of Triphala. Used for cleaning the eye.

(5) Daruharidra Kwath + Honey - For local application of eye.

(6) Daruharidra + Goat Milk - For local treatment.

(7) Til Tail - Sesame Oil.

Used in the form of Netra Basti.

Inflammatory Condition of eye : -

Sookshma Triphala - Orally 250 to 500 mg x 4 times daily.

[Reference : Intensive Training Programme for Australian Students, 1988]

Chapter : 22

Eyes in Upanishadas

Dr. P. N. Awasthi

चक्षुरेवर्गात्मा साम तदेतदेतस्यामृच्यध्यूढःसाम तस्मादृच्यूढःसाम गीयते। चक्षुरेव सात्मामस्तत्साम॥

'CHAKSHU' is 'RIK' and 'ATMA' is 'SAMA'. this way in this 'RIK ('CHAKSHU') 'SAMA' ('ATMA') is placed. Therefore, 'SAMA' which is placed in (part of) 'RIK' is sung. 'CHAKSHU' is 'Sa' and 'ATMA' is 'AMA'. Thus both combined are ''SAMA''.

'RIK' is supposed to be describable totality of knowledge and 'SAMA' is supposed to be the part of the totality used for singing the glory of 'DEVA'. Just as 'SAMA' is the part of 'RIK', Soul or life is the part of eyes, i.e. it is best reflected from the eyes or is best judged in the eyes. The word 'ATMA' here stands for 'CHHAYATMA', i.e. the reflected soul.

चष्टे = पश्यति अनेन इति चक्षुः

CHAKSHU' is that organ of sense through which one sees. It is obvious that unless mind and life are there the process of seeing, i.e. the process of visual perception does not take place. Eyes, therefore are the best sense organ for manifestation of life.

अथ यदेतदक्ष्णः शुक्लं भाः सैवर्गथ यन्नीलं परः

कृष्णं तन्साम। तदेतदेतस्यामृच्यध्यूढःसाम। तस्माद‍ृच्य–

ध्यूढ॰साम गीयते। अथ यदेवैतदक्ष्णः शुक्लं भाः
सैव साथ यन्नीलं परः कृष्णं तदमस्तत्साम।।

The white of the eye is 'RIK' and the black after the blue is 'SAMA'. In this way 'SAMA' is placed in 'RIK'. Therefore, 'SAMA' which is placed in 'RIK' is sung. The while of the eye is 'Sa' and the black after the blue is 'Ama' Thus both combined are 'SAMA'.

Shree Shankaracharya has commented that अथ यन्नीलं परःकृष्णे आदित्यइव दृक्शक्त्यधिष्ठनां तत्साम।

If Sun is seen with naked eyes it is seen as a blue disc with white periphery. Black disc is seen in the centre of the blue Sun disc because of its brightness and failure of our eyes to stand to it. This black spot persists in our visual field for some time afterwards also and gradually disappears. It appears, most of the corneas encountered in those days were blue. This also indicates the racial characteristics of the Indians of those days.

Whole of the eye – as such – is necessary for the anatomical and functional totality of the organ but the power of perception really lies in the centre and that is why it is to be praised.

अथ य एषोऽन्तरक्षिणि पुरुषो दृश्यते सैवक्तन्साम तदुक्थं तद्यजुस्तदब्रह्म। तस्यैतस्य तदेव रूपं यदमुष्प रूपं यावमुष्य रोष्णौ तौ. रोष्णौ यन्नाम तन्नाम।।

This 'PURUSH' seen in the eye along is 'RIK'. He is 'SAMA'. He is 'UKTHA'. He is 'YAJUH' and he is 'BRAHMA'. This 'PURUSH' of the eye has the same 'RUPA' as the one in the Sun. Whatever 'RAKSHAS' Sun has eye also has and whatever names Sun is given eye also is given. Shree Shankaracharya has commented on the word 'PURUSH'. 'पुरि = नगरे शयनात् पुरुषः' – 'पूश्यति वा स्वेनामना जगदिति पुरुषः'

one who lives in the town, i.e. in the body or one who fills up this world with his ownself is 'PURUSH'. First covers the body and second the world.

Eye and the Sun are taken to be similar here. The all pervaiding knowledge or the information force is present in both of them. The earlier three 'VEDA' ('RIK', 'SAMA' & 'YAJUH') deal with the same power at the level of ADHI DAIVAT'. i.e. its manifestation in the from of different 'DEVA', 'UKTHA' is 'OM' and 'BRAHMA' is the ultimate totality of power or energy. It is this who perceives through the eyes and appreciate the perceived in relevant contexts. It is this who showers energies from the Sun for every activity in this world.

These three 'MANTRAS' are taken from 'CHHANDOGYOPNISHAD'. From these 'MANTRA' the conclusions derived in order can be that –

1. Eyes are the wider source of information and they are the best indicator of life and conscious ('ATMA').

2. Eyes have white, blue and black parts and perception is done through the central most black part (Pupil), and

3. There is all pervaiding life or conscious force in the body or in the universe and it is this who perceives or knows.

The period of 'UPANISHADA' is supposed to be just after the 'VEDIC' period, but looking to the language, style and the expression it can be easily made out that some of the 'UPANISHADA' belong actually to the 'VEDIC' period. There are opinons but the least estimated period of 'VEDA' is 5000 years from now and 3000 years before Christ. The above stated 'MANTRA' just provide a glimpse of the knowledge prevalent in 'VEDIC' period in India.

I intend to discuss all the three conclusions in the light of modern knowledge briefly.

1. One of the greatest puzzle of the modern biology is to find out the secrets of the principles guarding the phenomena of 'Diversity and Integrity' at the same time. There are number of diversities in the growth from egg cell, yet the integrity is maintained even in the rebalious growth of malignant cells. They act within the body. If the diversity was not there we would not have seen the universe as it is. One million animals species and 2,65,500 species of plants would not be seen on our planet if there was no diversity. The diversity on the land has produced 93 per cent of the total number of species while marine species remain only 7 per cent, yet if the principle of 'unity of opposites' wasn't there, no individual will be formed including the masses of non-living matter – as we call them – the galaxies, the stars and the planets including the atoms – part of which possess opposite charges yet remain adherent together.

The first and the earlier living individual we know is the cell and the cell surely needs lot of information to survive. This information it gathers through its covering by direct contact. Information (ज्ञान) is supposed to be one of the very important ingredient in the process of evolution. No organisation can take place without information and any organisation leading to individuality has to be well informed. This is true not only for the living but for the non-living too.

Academician, V. M. Glushkov, wrote 'information exists because there are material bodies and, consequently, heterogeneities formed by them. Any heterogeneities formed by them. Any heterogeneity bears some information.' Word heterogeneity stands for separation, differentiation, recognition independent from the rest, and this is 'AHAM' (अहम्) factor the basis of analytical knowledge (विज्ञान) He further explains – "the stars for example, serve as a source of information by creating a certain heterogeneity in the distribution of substance and energy. The same is true of any object or phenomenon in the world around us. Thus organisation is a source of information. Since all the objects and processes of the world around us are, to some extent or an other connected together with different categories of links, they inevitably exchange not only substance and energy but also information." It amounts that the universe is full of substance and energy and they are full of knowledge.

A living individual has to be much more alert and informed to sustain its tiny individuality and one who is more informed and has better means of information only survives as the 'fittest'. The cellular multiplicity and complexity leads to complex tools for information not only for receiving but also for storing.

The most advanced and complex organism on the surface of this planet is the man and he is so because of the best tools he has, the senses, the memory, power of analysis and collaboration. We gather information from the world around us through five sense organs and they are just the tools.

"इन्द्रियेषु साथकतमत्वयोगात् कुठारवत्" –

2 / 39, 'SANKHYA DARSHAN'. (Since unavoidable add they are, for the external perception, senses are treated like an axe).

Two of the senses, eye and ear, have the wider range and between them eyes have the widest. It is calculated that 80 per cent of the total perception is accomplished through eyes. Eyes and ears catch up information from long distances but the range of eyes is the longest and finest. The olfactory sense is the medium range and touch and taste have the closest rnage, the actual contact. Eyes, therefore, are the best tool of information achieved by the organism in the process of evclution out of its efforts (कार्य) piled generation after generation.

Complex is built out of simple matter. "The beginning of the evolution of chemical compounds towards life dates from the moment when the crust was formed, i.e. about 4.5 thousand millions years ago. Consequently, the period of bio-chemical evolution, which ultimately led to the formation of the proto-organisms, is more than one thousand million years long." The earliest organism unearthed is 3100 million years old. It is estimated 'some 1200 million years ago, the biotic circulation accomplished previously by the single – celled organisms increased in complexity due to emergence of the multi cellular forms.' It was bout 400 million years ago that the preconditions were formed for the organisms to leave the water and populate the land. Life was thus not only born in water but was sustained in water only for nearly 2700 million years. It is for this reason, the word 'NARAYAN' is framed. NAR = Water, AYAN = Home. It was about 3.5 thousand million years ago that a single cell was formed and it still continues to be formed. Whether single or multiple, every cell has its own energy store, food store, internal information system and external information system and a permanent hereditary code system, etc. Thus cell is quite a complex entity and eyes are built out of very special cells for very special purpose.

Eye is most delicate and sophisticated organ, containing water part at the most. Eye is therefore, the delicate most indicator of life. Death we might be calling Brain Death, Heart Death or Lung Death, but it is best seen in the eyes. Dilated pupils and motionless glassy eyes are clear image of Death. The absence of life and consciousness – the 'ATMA'.

A full grown man is 60 per cent water by weight and a young one at the formative stage is 90 per cent water or even more. The muscles contains 76 per cent of water and heart 79.3 per cent.

The brain 83.3 per cent, but eyes contain water more than 90 per cent. Water has remakable temperature controlling capacities, because it has high heat capacity – high laten heat of fusion and evaporation – low heat conductivity and capacity for expansion before freezing. The eyes, therefore, can stand high heat but very high temperature harms them by altering their proteins. Extensive loss of fluid – severe dehydration – sinks the eyes and the vision is lost for every.

. It has been worked out that human body possesses as many cells as eighteen zeros in a row and they are utmost economically organised. Every cell in the body is a living one, and has its own entity. Yet, all of them fused together in supreme organisation indicate one life, one conscious and one entity. The total whole carrying the sense of oneness is the 'ATMA' in the body. This is the 'PURUSH' who receives all the informations.

We know that we possess convex lens in our eyes. Therefore, images falling over our retina must be up side down but we interprete them correctly and see the things as they are. It is experimentally seen that if the glasses are given to turn the images further upside down – the images are further corrected after some time automatically and correct interpretations are again achieved. It is also seen in many people that the visual perception – recognition of colour, shape, etc., can be accomplished through their fingers. Eyes not used for generations are lost. This seen in flies bred in dark for generations.

Animals living in peculiar conditions of nature develop suitable peculiar powers in their eyes. Eyes, therefore, are not that important. They are just tools modifiable as needed. Important is the 'ATMA' inside. it is on account of the 'ATMA' that senses make the senses. The 'ATMA', therefore, is to be praised.

2. The second 'MANTRA' only describes the visible eye. This is rather a better description than available in Ayurvedic Treatises. The 'NEEL = blue, is surely the colour of the iris and the black part is the pupil. The assignment of colours to 'BHUTA', white to 'JALA' and black to 'VAYU', etc., is too poetic an approach and it is surely under the influence of literary people handling Ayurveda. The 'UPANISHADA' presentation is just factual. The mention of blueness in the eyes indicates that 'UPANISHADA' are written in icy places, where eyes were blue commonly. As is described in 'VISHNU PURAN', 'BHARAT VARSHA' was named as 'HIMAVARSHA' earlier and this 'HIMAVARSHA' was the southern part of 'JAMBUDVIP'. India was thus more on Himalayas beyond Afghanistan and Caccasus, etc. 'Blue' eyes are still seen common in these areas. Light enters the pupils, was well known but perhaps nothing beyond was known as far as anatomy and physiology are concerned.

3. In the third 'MANTRA', eyes are very closely compared with 'the Sun. But the eyes are supposed to be only receiving instrument. And the Sun is supposed to be the donor of the energy. The whole of the energy cycle sustaining life in this world is initiated and maintained by the Sun. Out of all the sources of energy for this world – Sun, electric discharges,' cosmic rays, radioactivity and volcanos. Sun is the major most contributor. It provides radiation and ultraviolet rays in

different strengths. We know that most of the changes in the matter, including their properties, organic or inorganic, are carried out by changes in speeds and positions of electrons. Electrons are further activated by photons of the light of the Sun and that is how the whole life process goes on. Hungarian Biochemist Albertszent Gyorgyi has expressed that 'energy cycle of life consists of electrons being boosted up by photons, and then dropping back to their ground level through the living systems, giving up gradually their excess energy which then drives the living machinary. This way life is a continuous and regular cycle flow of electrons induced by the Sun radiation'.

Functionally eyes and the Sun are opposite to each other. Eyes are receivers and the Sun is the donor. But the investigations in the last ten to fifteen years in the bigger academies in U.S.S.R. & U.S.A. have proved with photographic evidences that every living body has an aura of energy around it and the energy can be made to flow out from fingers and palms of selected people. It can be pointedly made to flow out from eyes as well and it can be stored in containers. This energy has attracting powers even for the non-metalic substances and no matter can obstruct its action. Eyes—this way are not only receivers but also the projectors of the inborn energy. This is not a common process but it is systematised now. India has known and practised it for the ages together in the form of 'TRATAK', etc. The energy pointedly flowing out from the eyes is obviously generated in the body. Out of the five senses only two, i.e. eyes and skin are competent instruments for such out flow. So, eyes can behave also like the Sun, the donor. Now, the question arises, that if eyes and the Sun are similar, does the Sun receive the information like eyes? There is not scientific grounds for it to believe, except the general principle – stated earlier – that – all the masses being heterogenous do receive information. If the Sun is an eye – the receiving instrument – it must belong to the ultimate all knowing entity. We seek intelligence from him in 'GAYATRI MANTRA' – the eternal song for protection of the universe – 'GAYA'. = Song, 'TRI' = Protector when pray 'SAVITUH VARENYAM' 'superior to the Sun.'

Since upliftment of the individual human soul is the basis of the Indian Philosophies, and since souls are reflected in the eyes – eyes are given utmost important in the ancient Indian literature. The systematic study of the ancient Indian literature in the light of the modern sciences can provide a fascinating study with many practical hypothesis for the future investigations and understandings. Here is provided only a sample.

Whatever is stated in volumes nowadays is stated very briefly in these 'MANTRAS' in a fashion prevalent in those days. The present details available in the form of ophthalmic anatomy, etc., is just the continuation of the same knowledge and nothing separate or antagonistic. It is very much regrettable in India this knowledge is not fused but is kept arrested in a separate compartments.

In Indian literature, eyes are given very important position and are praised for the health and beauty all the while. But they are useless without sight. Eyes, therefore, must be protected. The eyes of our children are the eyes of our Nation and the Souls behind they are the Soul of Nation. Let us build them healthy.

Dr. P. N. Awasthi, Retd. Surgeon,
M.A. Podar Hospital, Bombay
&
Chief Editor, JNIMA.

Chapter :23

"A Study of Anti-Timira

(Anticataract)

Activity Of Katak (Strychnos Potatorum)"

Dr. Samir Kumar Pan,
Dr. J. M. Sharma,
Dr. M. K. Sevak (Jamnagar)

INTRODUCTION

We research scholars are indebted to the society. So we are bound to return something, for which they are waiting day after day. Before starting any research we have to keep in mind few rods :

1. is the topic, a burning problem to the society?
2. can research serve cheeper remedy?
3. is research much expensive?

Here the research topic is, study of anti-cataract activity by medicine, Katák. Blindnessia disability whose severity only the blind persons know, other persons can feel for them but can do nothing to mitigate their mental agonies and sufferings. According to W.H.O reports there are 10 to 15 million blind in the world. The latest survey carried out by the I.C.M.R. puts the number of blind in our country at 9.5. million, of these 70% are due to cataract. 10% due to glaucoma, 10% due to corneal diseases and remaining 10% are due to various disease. It has been calculated that unless dicisive action is not taken the population of the blind will be doubled in another 25 years.

Grimly aware of the sad situation the Govt. of India has launched N.P.C.B. (National Programme for Control of Blindness) programme. Not only India Govt. but the W.H.O. also took up the matter with utmost seriousness which was evident from its slogan "Foresight prevent blindness."

In this research, experimental study was not undertaken, since Katakseed is non-toxic as mentioned in various books viz. i) Indigenious drug by Chopra, ii) Wealth of India, iii) Kirtikar and Basu etc. and is also used in various Ayurvedic classics such as Charaka, Sushruta, Vagbhata, Yogaratnakara, Sharangadhara, Chakradatta and many Nighantus.

DURG PROFILE (Katak)

History - Description of Katak is not available in Atharvaveda. It is mentioned in Charak, Sushruta and Kashyapa Samhita. Sushruta has mentioned it among seven Jalaprasadana Dravyas. Not only that it is mentioned by Palakapya Samhita. It is also available in Harita, Bhela and many Nighantus like Rajanighantu, Dhanvantari Nighantu, Bhava Prakash, Shaligram etc.

Identification and Nomenclature : In ancient times, identification was mainly done by organoleptic method or by observing therapeutic action. Before Morphological description is not available in any Ayurvedic classic, in these ciricumstances the 'Katak' is identified from its Paryayas mentioned in various classics. Some of them are mentioned here Ambyprasadam, Katakam, Guchhaphala, Chakshushyam, Chhedaniya, Nirmalam, Netraprasada, Netravikarajit, Lekhanatmakam, Shodanatmakam etc. In modern it is identified by the following description of the plant.

A moderate size glabrous tree attaining 13 m. black bark, trunk often irregularly fluted, plentiful in deciduous forests of West Bengal, central and South India upto 12000 m.

Leaves - elliptic, 5-12 cm. long, 2.5 - 5 cm. breadth, acute, nearly sessile, glabrous and shining, 3 or 5 nerved.

Flowers - rather large for the genus, nearly sessile cymes. Calyx 2 mm. long, 5 segments, ovate acute corolla - 4.6 mm. long, 5 lobed oblong acute, stamen carpel 1 or 2.

Fruit - berry black when ripe 1.7 cm. diam. seeds - 1 or 2 circular 8 mm. diam. bluntly lenticular.

On the basis of morphological description this plant is taken under the family - Loganiaceae and named as Strychnos potatorum.

Classification :

in Modern

Div	Phanerogam
S. Div	Angiosperm
Class	Dicotyledon
S. Class	Gamopetalae
Series	Bicarpellatae
Order	Gentianales
Fa	Loganiaceae
Genus	Strychnos
Species	Potatorum

In Ayurveda it is classified by various authors in various ways.

1. Charaka	Madhura Skanda, Visagna Dasemani.
2. Sushruta	Parusakadigana, Madhura Varga, Galaprasadana Dravya.

3. As. Hr.	Parusakadiigana
4. Dhanvantari Nighantu	Chandandi varga
5. Raja Nighantu	Amradi varga
6. Shaligram Nighantu	Phala varga

Drug Analysis :

Loss on drying at 110°C	8.81% w/w
Ash Value	0.92% w/w
Acid insoluble ash	0.0971% w/w
Water soluble extractive	13.27% w/w
Alcohol soluble extractive	1.57% w/w
Volatile oil content	Nil
P^{H}	5.44

Pharmacological :

For clearing muddy water - it is due to the combined action of colloids and alkaloids in the seed. The albumin and other alkaloids sensitize the suspension and the coagulation is then caused by the alkaloidal iom. (Wealth of India, Vol. X).

Stomatic. demulcent and emetic properties and are used diarrhoea, diabetes, gonorrhoea and eye diseases. It is also used as a substitute for ipecac in the treatment of dysentry and bronchitis (Wealth of India Vol. X)

Ayurvedic pharmacological properites differ from each other in various classics.

1. Kaideva Nighantu	-	Tuvarana, Tikta, Vishada, Shitala, Laghu, Vikashi, Cheedi, Chakshusha, Kapha Vata nut.
2. Dhanvantari Nighantu	-	Tikta, Shitala, Mridu.
3. Bhava prakasha	-	Tuvarana, Madhura, Shitala, Guru.

4. Rajanighantu - Katu, Tikta, Ushna.

Disease Aspect :

The word 'Timira' means indistinct vision. According to Amarakosha the meaning of 'Timira' is darkness. Form the etymological derivation it is clear that 'Timira' means loss of light perception or darkness or blindness, which is the late stage of 'Timira Roga.'

Definiation of Cataract :

Cataract may be simply defined as denoting and opacity in the lens. Galen's (131-210 A.D.) conception was that the diseases lay in the brain and the visual nerves, whereas our Hindu medicine clearly mentioned that cataract is a diseases of the lens.

Aetiology to Timira :

Causes in general mentioned for all eye diseases are the causes of 'Timira' This disease has been mentioned as symptom or sequelae of some other diseases in the Ayurvedic texts.

A. General Causes :

• Excessive or deficient or wonderful use of the senses (Ch. Su. 11/39-41).

• Viruddha Ahara, Diwaswapna, Vega Nigraha, Atimaithuna.

• Intake of Ushna, Atikshara and Katu food items, injury, looking at fine objects, are the causative factors (Harita).

• Excessive or deficient oil bath, working with shaking hand, witch caraft, drug addiction, heavy weight lifting, looking at bright illuminating objects like sun, gems, gold or hot iron etc. (Netra Prakashika).

B. Specific causes of 'Timira' :

• After Ati Raktasrava (Su. Su. 14/30).

• Trauma to Avarta and Apanga Marmas (Su. Sh. 6/28).

• Grahani Roga (Ch. Chi. 15/61).

• Nasya Karma to a patient of fever, after the intake of alcohol (Ch. Sl. 9/115)

• Constipation and suppression of natural urges (Bhela Samhita Su. 6/6).

Aetiology of Cataract :

At the present time no complete and satisfying description can be given of the aetiology of cataract. Fundamentally the loss of transparency is due to a distrubance of lens fibres which form a colloid system into which a large amount of water is bound. The distrubance may be of two types (1) Swelling opacity - producing defective fibres, (2) coagulative opacity - chemical changes whereby the proteins become coagulated and insoluble. There are various causes for the formation of cataract. Senility, trauma, memtabolic, disturbance, toxic agent, due to infection, drug etc.

Samprapti of Timira and Lakshana (Symptom)

Nija Nidan Agantuja Nidan

Dosa Sanchaya

Continuation of Nidan Sevana

Prakopa

Diffusion of Dosas all over
the body through Siras and Srotas.

Prasara

Ascend of Doshas to Urdhvaja
fnigata part.

Sthana Samshraya

Localisation of Doshas in Patal

Drishti and Roopavaha Sira

Production of prodromal symptoms

Vyakta

1st Patala - Avyakta Darshana

2nd Patala - Vihwal Darshana

3rd Patala - Gochar Vibhrama (colouring of Drishti)

4th Patala - Linganasha

Pathology of Cataract :

Since the len is composed of single epithelial cells and fibres derived from them, no matter that the aetiology or type of cataract may be, the general pathological changes are essentially the same–degeneration of the lenticular fibres either of sclerosis or necrosis.

(1)Scierosis changes – due to some alternation in the permeability of the lens capsule, some of the cortical matter goes out and is absorbed. The lens becomes flatter, the capsule becomes thick.

(2)There is hydration due to accumulation of water droplets inbetween the fibres, followed by changes in the colloid system within the fibres. The proteins are first denatured and then are coagulated forming opacity.

Types :
1. Vataja Timira
2. Pittaja Timira
3. Kaphaja Timira
4. Raktaja Timira

5. Sannipataja Timira
6. Parimalayi Timira

Types of senile cataract :

1. Cortical cataract.
2. Nuclear /head cataract.
3. Posterior cortical/post sub cataract.

Clinical Study

Materials and Methods :

The patients for the study were taken from the outpatient department of I.P.G.T. & R., Jamnagar as well as from Dr. Sevak's Eye Hospital, Jamnagar.

After a brief ophthalmic and systemic history, best corrected vision was recorded.

Dilatation of pupil with 5% phenylephrine eye drops, the opthalmoscopic and retinoscopic examination was done.

If any opacity was present, if was classified and graded on a separate printed proforma.

No special colours are used as each subtype of opacity is drawn separately.

Whose pupil did not dilate or contraindicated were excluded from the study.

Only senile cataract was taken for the study.

Patients having vision 6/60 or better were included in this study.

Follow up patients at monthly intervals. Minimum follow up of 1 year was planned.

Age, sex, best corrected vision, cortical opacity extent, nuclear opacity extent, PSC opacity extent and ophthalmoscopically graded opacity extent are recorded.

The eye with more advanced cataract received topical

application of 'Katak' while the contralateral eye served as control. 37 immature cataract patients had been treated with 'Katak' of them 21 patients have completed the follow up of 3 months course or more. Katak used as a Anjana three times daily.

Follow Up :

The same steps of examination are repeated on the separate sheet without referring to the previous records.

The best corrected visual acuity is recorded at each follow up.

Discussion :

The studies were not double blind. We recognise this major pitfall but fell that because at teach follow up previous records were not referred, the bias is lessened.

Very few patient completed 1 year follow up treatment. Significant number of patients completed three months follow up, they were included for data analysis. Thus follow up ranges from 3 months to 1 year.

A very large drop out rate is possible explained by the fact of the patient learning that cataract can be surgically cured, from other ophthalmologists.

Pure type of cataract may turn to mixed type. Then it is difficult to corelate whether it is the preservation of vision, reduction in the speed of visual loss or the effect on extent of the opacity that is responsible for the improved vision. Pure type of cataract is minimum. Mixed typed are more common.

About Pharmacological action :

Katak has Shophaghna activity (Kd. N.) So it acts on intumation stage of cataract and cortical type soft cataract and PSC as Katak having Kaphanashaks, Lekhana and Chhedi property and Ushna Guna (by Raja Nighantu).

Katak is having Lekhaniya, Chhedaniya, and Laghu Guna so it acts also in sclerotic type and nuclear type of cataract.

According to aetiology of cataract, protein in lens becomes coagulated and insoluble. Due to it's Kashaya Rasa and Shita Guna the coagulated suspended proteins and settled down and a clear transparnet zone appears. Katak contains colloids and albumin like alkaloids, by combined action of these the coagulated suspended protein are settled down.

Conclusion :

1. Katak acts on three types of clinically divided senile cataract. It is more effective on cortical and lental sclerosis but not so in P.S.C.

2. From the study it is evinced that 'Katak seed' not only checks the progression of opacity but infact clears the lens also. This is explained by the fact that in the studied cases the vision showed marked improvement rather than remaining static.

To out pleasant surprise we could note that a few cases the vision was improved within one month of commencing the treatment.

Parameter	Discription
Patients	21
Male / Female	8/13
Age (years)	31-80
Follow up (months)	3-12

Type of cataract	No. of years.
Cortical	14
Nuclear	20
PSC	8
Total	22

Age Gr.	F	M	Total
34-40	1		1
41-50	2		2
51-60	6	4	10
61-70	4	2	6
71-80		2	2
Total	13 (61.9%)	8 (38.07%)	21

Vision	Cortical		Nuclear		Pse		Total	
	BT	**AT**	**BT**	**AT**	**BT**	**AT**	**BT**	**AT**
6/60	1	1	2		4	0		
6/36	3	1	5		1	2	9	3
6/14	3	1	4	3	1	1	8	5
6/18		2		1		1	0	4
6/12		3		6			0	9

CONTROL GR.

Vision	Cortical		Nuclear		Pse		Total	
	BT	**AT**	**BT**	**AT**	**BT**	**AT**	**BT**	**AT**
6/60	1	4	3	6	2	4	6	14
6/36	4	3	5	4	2		11	7
6/24	2		2				4	
6/18								

N.B.

Snellen's Chart Reading	Efficiency %
6/6	100
6/9	91.5
6/12	83.6
6/18	64.0
6/24	48.09
6/36	20.00
6/60	0.0

FFICIENCY % OF VISION

Catract		X ± SD	SE	t	P
Cortical	Control	8.57 ± 10.69	0.38	6.20	<0.001
	Treated	63.84 ± 23.60	8.92		
Nuclear	Control	8.00 ± 10.33	3.26	19.26	<0.001
	Treated	70.99 ± 16.92	0.32		
PSC	Control	0 ± 0	0	3.49	<0.05
	Treated	38.02 ± 21.80	10.90		

AREA % OPACTY

Catract		X ± SD	SE	t	P
Cortical	Control	56.86 ± 9.65	3.65	6.45	<0.001
	Treated	22.86 ± 10.07	3.81		
Nuclear	Control	55.9 ± 7.89	2.5	10.08	<0.01
	Treated	19.4 ± 8.28	2.62		
PSC	Control	63.75 ± 2.5	1.25	5.54	<0.01
	Treated	34.00 ± 10.46	5.22		

[Reference : Ayurveda Education Series - 40 Musing Ayurveda : Editor - P. H. Kulkarni - 1992]

[- Inernational Seminar on Ayurveda]

Chapter : 24

Ocular manifestations in diabetes & its relation to constituion (Prakruti)

Dr. S. M. Sathye

Aetiology & Symptoms

Diabetes mellitus is a disease of metabolism which is characterized by a failure of the tissues of the body to oxidise carbo-hydrates at the normal rate. This future is due to lack of insulin.

In the aetiology of diabates, a disease cheefly of middle life, heredity, obesity and sacial susceptibility are important predisposing factors.

The following symptoms point to diabetes mellitus :

Fasting Blood Sugar Level above 120, P. P. Blood Sugar after meal above 180.

Manifestations :

Diabetes is known to cause Ocular manifestations. The manifestations are as follows :-

(1) Changes in the refraction : Increase in blood sugar is supposed to be accompanied by a decrease in refraction manifested by an increase in hyperopia (Hypermetropia).

(2) Accommodation and ocular muscles : The ability to use the eyes for close work may become impaired in some patients because of a weakened conition of the accomodation.

(3) Ocular muscle palsy : The sixth nerve is the most frequently affected, with the imparied action of external rectus muscle that leads to diplopia.

(4) Diabetic inties

(5) Cataract.

(6) Glaucoma.

(7) Diabetic retionopatiy

(8) Lipemia Retinalis.

Notes on the above

Out of all the above complications cataract, diabotic retinopathy, occular muscle palsy, and disturbance in acesmmodation are commonly soon while the other complications are comparatively rare.

It has also been observed that the blood sugar level at any time bears no definite relationship to the occurrence of eye lesions. But the aetiology of eyemamfestations they have some relation to the (1) age, (2), use of insulin and (3) frequent change in blood sugar levels.

But it has been found that usually eye manifestations develop after about ten years of diabetes. They are usually common in long-standing cases of diabets.

On observing such long-staning cases of diabestes, it is found that in some we get retinal change in some cataract, an in some palsy.

I have observed 50 long-standing cases of diabetes. It is surprising that not all the symptomes are manifested in all.

In some there are haemorrhage but no cataract; In some there is cataract but no haemorrhage; in some there is ocular palsy but no cataract or any retinal change.

(1) When the patient has been suffereing from the same disease for 20 years he should display all the symptoms. If he does not we should seek the reason

therefor. Can we explain why we get harmorrhage in one, cataract in another and palsy in the third?

(2) Another point is whether we can speculate about the type of comlications in a particular patient; if we could, we will be able to prevent the complications by giving suitable drugs. According to the information available in modern science, we cannot speculate what sort of complications a particular diabetic patient will develop.

While studying the cases of ocular complications in diabetes, I observed that we can solve the problem by Ayruvedic principles.

Ocular complications studied in depth :

The inference from the data collected by me are as follows : (1) A patient of Kaphaja constitution usually develops cataract. (2) A patient of Pittaja constitution usually develops retinal changes or retinal complications. (3) A patient of Vataja constitution usually develops occular muscle palsy or Glaucoma.

Conclusion :

. I think this information we glean by studying the constitution of the patient tells us of his prononess to a particular type of complication and is very useful in guiding him to avoid the factor which may load to the complications.

The study of the Constitution is hence a must whenever a diabetic patient comes to a physician or an opthalmologist.

Patients of mixed constitution have mixed ocular complications. I have given a detail information to find of the constitution of a patient.

From the information given below. One can find out the constituion of a patient according to Ayurvedic point of view & he will be able to speculate about the possible ocular complications in a diabetic patient.

If the constitution is known we definitely prevent the possible complications in a diabetic patient by giving suitable aurvedic drugs.

My experience about the treatment & now I could avoid the complication will be given in the text issue.

I would like to request all the readers to collect a data accordingly.

This information will definitiely help the ophthalmologist & the physicians while treating the cases of diabetes.

1. Kapha Prakruti :

Kapha, being unctuous, those of Kapha habitus have glossy limbs, on account of its smoothness they have smooth limbs, owing to its softness they have pleasent, delicate and clear bodies, owing to its sweetness they have profuse semen, desire for sex-act, and children on account of its firmness, they have firm, well knit an stable bodies, owing to the denseness of Kapha, they are plump and rounded in all their bodies and limbs. Owing to its slowness, they are slow in their actions and speech, due to its stability, they are slow in their undertakings and in the change of moods and pathological condition. Owing to its heavy-ness they are of firm, large and stable gait, owing to its coldness, their hunger thirst heat and persperation are meagre. Owing to its viscidity, they are firm and wellknit in their joints. Similarly owing to its clearness they are of clear looks, of clear and mellow complexion an voice.

Owing to the combination of such qualities those of Kapha habitus are possessed of strength, wealth, knowledge, vitality gentleness and long life.

2. Pittaja Prakruti :

Pitta is a hot, acute, fluid, raw, meatish in smell, acid and pungent.

Owing to its, those of Pitta habitus are intolerant of heat, very hot in the mouth of delicate and clear bodies, and have profuse moles, freckles, spots, pimples, on the body, excessive hunger and thirst are subject to early wrinkles, grayhair and boldness and are possessed generally of scanty, Soft and tawny hair on the head face and body. Owing to its acuteness they are possed of keen valour and acute digestive fire are given to taking excersive quantity of food and drink are subject to incapacity to bear suffering an are conconstant enters. Owing to its fluidity they have flabby and soft joints and flesh and profuse discharge of sweat, urine and faeces. Owing to its rawmeatish smell, they smell very much in their armpits; mouth, head, body, Owing to its pungant and acid taste, they a have small quantity of semen, limited sex appetite, and scanty offspring.

Owing to a combination of such qualities those of Pitta habitus are of moderate strength, and life span and moderate knowledge, experience wealth and means.

3. Vataja Prakruti :

Vata is dry, light, unsteady, abundant, swift, cold, rough and clear.

Owing to its dryness, those of Vata habitus are of dry wasted and small bodies of long drawn dry low broken hallow and horse voice, and are always weakful Owing to its lightness they are light and inconstent of gait, behaviour, diet, speech, owing to its unsteadiness they are restless in their joints, eyes, brows, jaws, lips, tongues, heads, shoulders, hands and feets. Due to its abunance, they are given to much talk and have prominent veins and tendons. Owing to its swiftness they are quick in their undertakings and variation of moods an pathological changes. They are quickly affected by fear likes and dislikes. They are quick in grasping and in forgetting too. Owing to its cold quality they are intolerant of cold and are gratey liable to suffer cold, shivering and stiffness. Owing to its roughness, they are rough hair on the head face and body, rought nails, teeth, rough mouth, hands & feet. Owing to its clearness they have cracked limbs and their joints always make noise as they walk.

Owing to the combination of such qualities those have vath habitus are generally of small strength, short lifespan, scanty off-spring and means and of meagre wealth.

In combine habitance the qualities also combine.

[International Conference on Ayurveda & Diabetes. 2003]

Chapter : 25

Role of Paripathadi Kwath In Karn-Srav (Otitis Media)

Dr. Ashok G. Wali

Introduction :

In my daily practice I get many patients having problems of KARNSRAV, mainly in chilren. Parents are also worried about KARNSRAV and complain regarding use of ear-rops prescribed. It is said that these ear-drops provide the temporary relief and not complete cure of the disease. This disease has multiple causitive factors.

I think in modern medicine they use only antibiotics and in some cases they suggest surgical work. In this connection to help this social problem I have decided to study the KARN-SRAV cases.

I found D.K. Sandu's patent production called Paripathadi Kadha which may help in these cases. Therefore I have chosen the topic for the paper - Role of Paripathadi Kadha in KARN-SRAV (Otitis-Media).

Ayurvedic Concept :

In Ayurveda the Karn-Roga is highly discussed. The number of Karn-Roga is different in various granthas.

There are many organic causes according to Ayurveda for KarnSrav. But for the sake of project I had selected only those patients who were having history of Hyperpyrexia, Measles, Chiken Pox and Jaundice as a root-cause.

In various types of Jwar (Fever) only in Arun Jwar (Scarlet fever) having a symptom like Karn-Srav. This is stated in Atharva-Veda.

But there is no any symptom like Karn-Srav in Measles, Chiken pox and Jaundice.

Vd. Atmaramshastri Datar has referred, "the effect of various diseases mainly measles, small-pox, chicken pox, having the symptom of high grade fever, which badly affects the organ Karn (Ear)".

Accordingly the Panchamahabhoot Sidhanta, (Five grass elements theory) Tej (hot) mahabhoot is increased which decreases the Akash (Space) and Vayu (Air) mahabhoots. Tej mahabhoot having hot property so it affects also the Apa (water) and Prithvi (earth) mahabhootas. Because of this effect of Tej mahabhoota, ear begins to flow which is known as Karn-Srav.

Materials and Methods

(A) MATERIAL :-

PARIPATHADI KADHA D. K. SANDU'S PATENT MEDICINE WAS DESIRED DRUG FOR THE TRIAL.

PARIPATHADI KADHA

Contains :-

1.. PARIPATH : - OLDENLANDIA HERBACEA ROXB. HORT.

2. GULABKALI : - ROSA CENITIFOLIA LINN.

3. RAKTACHANDAN:- PETEROCARPUS-SANTALINUSLINN.

4. YASTIMADHU :- GLYCHYRRHIZA GLABRA LINN.

5. GUDUCHI :- TINOSPORA CORDIFOLIA (WILD)
6. MANUKA :- VITIS VINIFERA LINN.
7. BALHIRDA :- TERMINALIA CHEBULA RETZ.
8. BRAHMAI :- CENTELLA ASIATICA (LINN) URBAN.
9. HALADI :- CURCUMAL LONGRA LINN.
10. SONAMUKHI :- SENNA
11. ADULASA :- ADHATODA VASCIA NEES.
12. DHANE :- CORIANDRUM SATIVUM LINN.
13. PITTAPAPADA :- FUMARIA VAILLANTI LOISEL
14. JIRE :- CUMINUM CYMINUM LINN.
15. KADU PATOL :- TRICHOSANTHES DIOICA ROXB.
16. DHAMASA :- FAGONIA CRETICA LINN.
17. KHAIRSAL :- ACACIA CATECHU WILLD
18. MUSTA :- CYPERUS ROTUNDUS LINN.
19. KHAS :- VETIVERIA ZIZANIODIS (LINN) NASH.
20. KADE CHIRAYATA :- SWERITA CHIRAYITA KARST.
21. NIMB :- AZADIRACHTA INDICA A. JUSS.
22. KUTAKI :- PICRORHIZA KURROA ROLYEEX BENTH.
23. GHATAKI :- WOODFORDIA FRUTICOSA KURZ.

(for fermentation)

(B) Methods :

Patient having history of Hyperpyrexia, Measles,

Chiken pox and Jaundice were selected for this disease. They were given medicine a trial drug - Paripathadi Kadha - D. K. Sandu's patent product.

Desired dosage was as follows :-

	Age Group	Dosage
A)	Infants	1/2 T.S.F. B.D.
B)	1 Year - 5 Years	1 T.S.F. B.D.
C)	6 Years - 15 Years	2 T.S.F. B.D.
D)	16 Years & Onwards	2 T.S.F. B.D.

No any dietery restrictions were advised upto 5 years. But above 5 years I have advised them to avoid chilly.

Partents were advised to clean the ear with hot water and put the swab in the ear.

The treatment was continued upto 90 days and follow up was observed after every 15 days.

Discussion :

It is observed that the high grade fever affects the organ-ear in Hyperpyrexia, measles and chiken pox.

There is no any symptom like fever in jaundice but according to Ayurveda this disease is of 'Pittavikar' Pitta dosha and Rakta dhatu has an ashray - ashrayee Bhav (inner independent) so Rakta Dhatu (Blood) impuredy by Pitta dosha means Ushna guns of Pitta increases ushna guna in Rakta (Blood) which circulates throughout the body ultimately this ushna guna affects the organ - ear.

Looking in to all ingradients Paripathadi Kadha is considered to be good "Pittaghna" dravyas (drugs).

The Guna (property) of this dravyas (drugs) is Laghu (light) and Rukhsa (Rough) which increases the Akash and Vahu mahabhootas. The Rasa (Test) is Tikta (Astringent) and Kashaya (Bittar) which reduce the watery discharge or pus and this increases 'Vata' so ultimately it decreases

'Pitta'.

The 'Veerya' (Potency) is sheet (cold) so this decreases the ushna guna (hot property) of disease.

Therefore it may help to improve the condition in Karn-Srav.

Statistical Data :

Totally 44 trial patients were treated, out of that 13 were dropped out. Therefore 31 patients were counted as hundred percent.

Chart - 1

Patients according to Age groups

Age	Male	Female	Total
A) Infants	01 (03.22%)	00 (00.00%)	01 (03.22%)
B) 1 to 5 Years	06 (19.35%)	04 (12.90%)	10 (32.25%)
C) 6 to 15 Years	09 (29.03%)	08 (25.80%)	17 (54.83%)
D) 15 & Onwards	02 (06.45%)	01 (03.22%)	03 (09.67%)
Total	18 (58.05%)	13 (41.92%)	31 (99.99%)

Chart - 2

Patients according to History wise.

Age	High Fever Chiken Pox			Measles			Jaundice			Total
	Male	Female	Total	Male	Female	Total	Male	Female	Total	
Infants	01	00	01	00	00	00	00	00	00	01
1 to 5 Yrs.	05	04	09	01	00	01	00	00	00	10
6 to 15 Yrs.	03	02	05	05	06	11	01	00	01	17
16 & Onwards	00	00	00	01	01	02	01	00	01	03
Total	09	06	15	07	07	014	02	00	02	31

	Male	Female
A) Hyperpyrexia	50.00%	46.15%
B) Measles	38.89%	53.85%
C) Jundice	11.11%	00.00%
Total	100.00%	100.00%

Chart - 3

Reatment according to AGE GROUPS.

Age	Best Results			Moderate Results			No Results			Total
	Male	Female	Total	Male	Female	Total	Male	Female	Total	
Infants	00	00	00	01	00	01	00	00	00	01
1 to 5 Years	02	02	04	04	02	06	00	00	00	10
6 to 15 Years	06	03	09	03	04	07	00	01	01	17
16 & Onwards	01	01	02	01	00	01	00	00	00	03
Total	09	06	15	09	06	15	00	01	01	31

	Male	Female
Best Results	50.00%	46.15%
Moderate Results	50.00%	46.15%
No Results	00.00%	7.70%
Total	100.00%	100.00%

TOTAL RESULTS

Best Results 48.38%

Moderate Results 48.38%

No Results 3.22%

Analysis :

According to statistical data we can anaylses the following points :-

1) There were more males (18) than females (13)

2) Maximum patients were of age group 6 to 15 years (17) followed by 1 to 5 years (10).

3) Number of males and females were likely to be equal in age group 6 to 15 years.

4) There were best results - 48.38% and moderate results also 48.38%.

5) There were 03.22 patients who showed no results.

6) In males Best and Moderate results were equal i.e. 50%.

7) In females Best and Moderate results were equal i.e. 46.15%.

Criteria's of Results

(A) Best Results	:	No Karn-Srav within 30 days and thereafter.
(B) Moderate Results	:	No Karn-Srav after 31 days to 90 days.
(C) No Results	:	If the Karn-Srav is unchanged after 90 days of treatment.

Conclusion :

Almost 48.38% Best and 48.38% Moderate results suggerst that Paripathadi Kadha has the Potency to improve Karn-Srav within ninty days, in patients having history of high grade fever, measles, chiken pox and jaundice.

No major side effects are observed.

ACKNOWLEDGEMENT :

MY GURU

Vd. Atmaramshastri Datar

MY COLLEAGUES

Dr. Vivek Hatadavanekar

Dr. (Mr. & Mrs.) Suru.

MY SPECIAL THANKS :

Prof. S. A. Kumbhar

Mr. S. B. Patil

Mrs. & Mr. Aba Datar

and

All members of Panchbhautik Chikitsa and Research Centre, Sangli.

BIBLIOGRAPHY

1) Current Diagnosis and Treatment

By Henry Brainerd, Sheldon Margen, Milton Chatton Published

by Large Medical Publication Los Altos, California 1963.

2) Sushruta Samhita

Published by Chaukhambha Sanskrit Sansthan Varanasi (1977).

3) Charaka Samhita

Published by Chaukhambha Sanskrit Sansthan Varanasi (1977).

4) Sartha Vagbhata

By Dr. Garde 7th edition 1983 published by Gajanan Book Depot, Bombay.

5) Yogaratnakara

Edited by Bhisagratna Brahmasankar Sastri Published by Chaukhambha Sanskrit Sansthan Varanasi, 3rd Edition 1983.

6) Kaya-Chikista

By Ram Raksha Pathak Vol. II Published by Chaukhambha Sanskrit Sansthan Varanasi, 2nd Edition 1979.

7) Panchbhautik Chikitsa & Balroga

By Vd. A. V. Datar, published by Mr. V. P. Datar, Sangli, First Edition 1988.

8) Panchbhautik Chikitsa Part - I

By Vd. A. V. Datar, published by Mr. V. P. Datar, Sangli, 2nd Edition 1990.

9) Dravyaguna Vijnana Vol. - II.

By Prof. P. V. Sharma, Published by Chaukhambha Sanskrit Sansthan Varanasi, 4th Edition, 1978.

10) Ayurveda Revisited
By Dr. Shardini A. Dahanukar and Dr. Urmila M. Thatte Published by Popular Prakashan, Bombay 1989.

[Reference : Ayurveda Education Series 40, 'Musing Ayurveda' Editor : P. H. Kulkarni 1992]

Chapter : 26

Concept of Nasya Karma In Shiro Rogas With Special Reference To Ardhavabhedaka And Its Management

By

Dr. Mrs. Lalitha B. R.

Guide : Prof. Dr. P. H. Kulkarni

Consists of following chapters.

I) Introducing

II) Review of Literature

1. Concept of Nasva Karma in Shiro rogas.
   a) Nasa Sharira - (Anatomy of Nose)
   b) Gandha Gnana - (Physiology of otfaction)
   c) Mechanism of action of Nasya
   d) Shiro rogas.
2. a) Aradhavabhedaka
   b) Migraine
   c) Trans Cranial doppler study (TCD)
3. Management of Ardhavabhedaka
   a) Nasya Karma
   b) Shiro Basti
   c) Anuvasana Basti
4. Review of ingredients selected in formulation

III) Material & Methods

a) Pharmaceutical Study

b) Phytochemical Study

c) Clinical Study

d) Trans Cranial doppler study (TCD)

IV) Observation

V) Discussion & Conclusion.

I) Introduction : Ashtanga Ayurveda highlights critical features for health & illhealth. The term shula is said to be derived from trishula of shiva, which causes severe pain or agony to mankind. Shula is a symptom which can affect any part, conventionally affects shiras also. Shriorogas are of 11 types, Ardhava bhedaka is one among them, which is the commonest prevalent problem is substantial minority of population affecting day to day activities of an individual. If timely therapeutic intervention is negleted, it results in grevious complications like loss of vision & hearing.

At the outset, with an insight to modern medical science, Ardhava bhedaka can be compared to Migraine, which is characterised by periodic, episodic, hemicranial, throbbing, pulsatile headache often accompanied by nausea and Vomitting. Though considered as disease previsouly, at present it is regarded as psychosocial problem / symptom. Shira Shula is said to be a symptom in various diseases and has been managed since earlier days. The enterprising part of management by our acharyas based on the quotation "Urdhwa Jatru Vikareshu Visheshan Nasya Mishyate" Nasya is beneficial in urdhwa jatru vikras as nose is the pathway to head, (Nasa hi shiraso dwaram) Nasya is effective in Shiro rogas hence to seek safe economical, cost effective remedy. An effort is made and being carried out by hypothesising that Nasya therapy eleminates vitiated doshas from shiras for this purpose the following ingredients were selected and formulated.

1. Shirisha - Albezzia lebbeck (seeds)
2. Apamarga - Achyranthes aspera (whole plant)
3. Mundi - Sphranthes indicus (whole plant)
4. Maricha - Piper nigrum (Fruits)
5. Guggulu - Commiphora guggulu (Gum)
6. Godanti - Calcium sulphate (CaSo4)

Treatment was categorised into 4 different groups to adopt better method of approach. 4 different groups were

1. Nasya - Sneha Nasya
2. Shamana Oushadhi
3. Shiro Basti
4. Anuvasana Basti

In first three groups, the formulation did not contain godanti (CaSo4 Calcium sulphate) and the igredients selected were kapha-vata shamaka in herbs and Godanti being Pitta Shamaka.

The present study has been planned to assess the efficacy of ingredients with supportive phyto chemical analysis, further the effect of the compound formulation is assessed by clinical study by adotping Trans cranial doppler study (TCD) as parameter. TCD - a non invasive ultra sound technique to assess cerebral blood flow in MCA (Middle cerebral artery)

II. REVIEW OF LITERATURE

a) "Concept of Nasya Karma in Shire rogas" Available and related literature high lighting Nasa Sharira (Anatomy of Nose), Gandha Gnana (Physiology of olfaction), Mechanism of action of Nasya, Shiro rogas are collected, reviewed critically to understand and analyse the concept of Nasya Karma.

2. a) Ardhava bhedaka - Recapitulation of Ardhava bhedaka, briefing about its nidana panchaka, vyavachedaka nidana, from briha trayee, laghu trayee and other texts.

b) Migraine - It is reviewed in detailed manner regarding its aetiopathogenesis with I.H.S. (International headache society) diognostic criteria.

c) Trans Cranial doppler study (TCD) - Technique is reviewed in detail.

4. Management of Ardhava bhedaka - Line of treatment is dealt in detail, with special reference to Nasya Karma, Shiro Basti and Anuvasana basti.

5. Review of Compound Fromulation - Extensive literary survey regarding selected ingredients of formulation is done.

III. MATERIAL AND METHODS :

a) Pharmacentical Study : - In the present study. The components of the formulation were studied in two forms 1) Capsules (2) Taila - The constituents selected viz. Apamarga, Shirisha, Mundi, Maricha, Purified, guggulu, were taken and powdered separately, made into homogenous mixture. Godanti (Caso4) was purified, incinarated mixed in equal proportion and made into capsules of 500 mg.Taila was prepared using same ingredeints except godanti basma, as per taila paka vidhi (Sha. M. k. h. 9 chapter.)

b) Phytochemical study :- The prepared formulations were analysed for physico chemical & phytochemical tests like alkaloids, saponins, tanins, steriods, gum and resins, were done to obtain consistent results.

Churna		**Taila**	
1.	Organoleptic	1.	Organoleptic
2.	Phytochemical	2.	Acid Value
3.	Loss on drying at 110°	3.	Refracticve index at 40°

4.	Ash Value	4.	Specific gravity
5.	Acid insoluble ash	5.	Ash value
6.	Alcohol soluble extractive	6.	Volatile content
7.	Water soluble extractive	7.	Saponification Value
8.	Thin Layer Chromatography (TLC) Investigation	8.	Un saponifiable matter
9.	Qualitative estimation of Ca. in Caso4.	9.	Peroxide Value
		10.	Thin Layer Chromatography (TLC Investigation)

c) CLINICAL STUDY :- The patients were selected randomly in the age group of 20-40 years with 2-4 years of chronicity, irrespective of sex, categorised into 4 groups viz.

Group - A	Sneha Nasya
Group - B	Shamana Oushadhi
Group - C	Shiro Basti
Group - D	Anuvasana Basti

30. Patients in each group were studied, diognosed as per case sheet proforma and taken up for line of management on the basis of subjective symptamatology and I.H.S. criteria. Treatment was given for 7 days and follow up was done for 3 months.

4. Trans cranial doppler study :-

Base line Trans cranial doppler study was done to fix the normal readings of cerebral blood flow in middle cerebral artery (MCA). Then TCD was done for patients during head ache attack within 48 hours and after 7 days of treatment to assess cerebral blood flow in MCA. Peak Systolic, End diastolic, Time average peak, Pulsatility index, resistivity index in cms/sec was recorded.

4. OBSERVATION :-

a) Pharmaceutial Study : It was noted that Godanti basma (calcium sulphate) was insoluble in prepared medicated oil.

b) Phytochemical Study : In this study the following observations in churna and taila were made.

CHURNA-ANALYTICAL FINDINGS.

1. Organoleptic	Colour - Pale Brown	
	Odour - Pungent	
	Touch - Coarse	
	Taste - Pungent	
2. Ph. 1% W/V solution		5.4%
3. Loss ond drying at 110°		8.641%
4. Ash Value		9.1
5. Acid insoluble-Ash		3.572
6. Alcohol Soluble extractive		30.166%
7. Water soluble extractive		20.025%

TAILA ANALYTICAL FINDINGS

1. Organoleptic	Colour - Brown	
	Odour - Stightly pungent	
	Texture - Oily	
	Taste - Slightly pungent	
2. Acid Value		5.7
3. Refractive Index at 40° C		1.4665
4. WT/ML Specific Gravity 20°C		0.9188

5. Saponification Value — 372.45
6. Un saponifiable matter — 0.24%
7. Volatile Oil — 0.1%
8. Peroxide Value — 4.22
9. Iodine Value — 55.7%
10. Ash Value — 0.12%

c) Thin layer chromatography : - The spots on TLC plates with reference to its Rf values for aqucous & methanol extracts were recroded.

3. IN CLINICAL STUDY :- In this study response to treatment was as follows, protocol was total relief, significant relief, slight relief, no relief.

	Significant relief	**Intensity of Pain Reduction**	**Post Ponement of Head Ache attack**
Nasya	highly significant	highly significant	moderate
Shamana Oushadhi	slight relief	moderately significant	significant
Shiro Basti	significant relief	significant relief	moderate
Anuvasana Basti	highly significant	moderate	highly significant

ऑगस्ट

4. Trans Cranial doppler study evaluates that Blood flow in middle cerebral artery is less at the time of head ache attack with in 48 hours and after treatment, blood flow in middle cerebral artery is increased.

DISCUSSION & CONCLUSION

On the basis of pharmaceutical phytochemical, clinical & Trans Cranial doppler study. The study can be conculded as follows.

1. Nasya, shamana oushadhi, shiro basti, Anuvasana basti are proved to be efficient in the management of Ardhava bhedaka.

2. Nasya has helped in reducing - acute intensity of head ache.

3. Shamana oushadhi is helpful as prophylatic measure.

4. Shiro basti is competent therapy to reduce intensity of pain in vata prakruti, tension and stress induced chronic patients.

5. Anuvasana basti has significantly helped in postponement of head ache attack. With reduction of intensity of head ache.

6. Trans cranical doppler study is better technique to evaluate cerebral flow in middle cerebral artery in migraine.

[Reference : International Seminar on Neurology, 2003]

Chapter : 27

Role of Vaman Karma in Shalakya Tantra

(Ear, Nose, Throat & Eyes)

1) EMESIS THERAPY :-

This is a process by which the contents of the stomach including kapha and pitta will be thrown out of the body through mouth. General concept of vaman means vomiting of the stomach contents.

It is Urdhwa Bhaga Shodhan. (Upper part purification)

According to Ayurveda, Shodhan treatment should be done with the way which is near to the Dushta Srotasa (Vitiated chanel) having 'Kha' Vaigunya (Vitiated part which gets affected by doshato create the diseases) of the ENT diseases. According to this rule for diseases related to Shalakya mouth is the nearest route, Hence Vaman is more applicable in ENT diseases.

2) ENT diseases in which Vaman is Indicated.

1) Peenasa (Rhinorrhoea)

2) Gala graha (Spasm of throat muscle)

3) Galaganda (Lymphadenitis)

4) Praseka (ptylism)

5) Hrillasa (Nausea)

6) Arochaka - (Anorexia)

7) Mukha paka (Stomatitis)

8) Other Urdhawa roga (other ENT diseases)

9) Netrabhishyanda (Conjunctivitis)

3) ENT diseased patients in which vaman is contra indicated :

1) Atisthoola (Obese)
2) Ati Krusha (Weak)
3) Ati Ruksha (Dry)
4) Vruddha (Old aged)
5) Balak (Children)
6) Garbhini (pregnant Woman)

7) Urdhawaga Rakta Pitta (bleeding from ear/nose/ throat, mouth)

8) Swar Upaghata (Disorders of voice)

9) Timira (Fainting)

10) Shir-shoola (Headache)

11) Karna Akshi shoola (Ear/Eye pain)

12) Bhrama (Giddiness)

4) PREPERATION :

For vaman karma, snehan karma and swedan karma should be done for 3 to 7 days.

Abhyantara sneha pana - Ghee or Til Tail (Seasame Oil) Ask the patients to drink per day in increasing quantity, for 3 to 7 days - Starting dose 25 to 50 ml. and increased by equal quantity.

During this period Bahya shehan + swedan is carried out to the patient.

When the signs of samyaka snehana (Proper oleation) observed snehana process should be stopped as follows-

1) Vatanulomya - (वातानुलोम्य) - Normal Vatadirection

2) Deeptogni - (दिप्तोग्नी) (अग्निवर्धन) Increase digestive power.

3) Asanhata Snigdha Varcha : stool - semi solid and with oil or ghee (वर्च स्निग्ध असंहत)

4) Sneha Udvega - Nausea to take sneha (स्नेह उद्वेग)

5) Klama - sleepiness. (क्लम)

Rukshana' (Create dryness) for one day patient is adviced to take only Bahya-shenhan + svedan Ati night patient is adviced to take Abhishandi (oozing) food (अभिष्यंदी आहार) for easy Vaman process.

5) PRE OPERATIVE PROCEDURE :

1) Collection of drugs/instruments 2) Examination of patients

3) Deciding dose of an emetic 4) Preparation of patient

6) COLLECTION OF DRUGS AND INSTRUMENTS :

Necessary Medicines :

Vaman Dravya - Madan Phal / Yastimadhu / Vacha / Kashmari / Saindhav (Rock salt) / Pippali (Piperlongum) Honey etc.

Instrument - Necessary pots to prepare kwatha (decoction) measuring cylinders - buckets, containers, towel etc.

7) EXAMINATION OF PATIENT :

1) Patient should be indicated for Vamana karma.

2) His Bala should be enough for Vaman Karma.

3) He should be good follower of instruction gives by Doctors.

4) According to Patient's -

(i) Vitiated Dosha / Dushya / Strength of disease (ii) Agni (iii) Satwa / Satmya (iv) Kostha (v) Age (vi) Time (vii) Country (viii) Prakrui,

These important points should be examined before advicing vaman Karma.

Then Abhyantara snehapana (internal oleation) swedana (Sudation) carried out to patients from 3 to 7 days upto sufficient sneha lakshana mentioned above.

1) During snehapana patients should drink hot water.

2) Patient should not sleep during day

3) He should take his normal food only when he has appetite.

4) Maithuna (sexual activity) Aatap sevan (hotatmosphere) Maruta sevan (cold environment) should be avoided.

By following these rules patient come under Samyaka sneha (proper oleation) symptoms within 3 to 7 days.

Then one day without giving Aabhyantara snehapana (internal oleation) only bahya snehan swedan (external sudation & oleation) be given to patient and adviced rest. By this remaining doshas travels to kostha (trunk) from shakta. (extremities). That night patient is adviced to take Abhishyandi.

Aahar like, Fish, masha, prepared food for utkesha of Doshas. (उत्क्लेष)

Next day early morning after sunrise patient prepared by. Bahya snehan, (external oleation) swedan (sweating) Patient should clear bowels and urine before doing vamana karma. Then Vamaka paste (chatan) (linctus) is prepared as follows -

Madan Phal + Honey + Pippali + saindhav (Rocksalt)

10 gm. + 20 gm + 5 gm. + 5 gm.

This paste should given to patient as the starter of vamankarma.

Then kwatha (decoction) of Yastimadhu (glyceriza) churna is prepared by standard methods. Patient is adviced to drink yastimadhu Qwath (decoction) upto Kantha (Throat).

Then we should wait for vaman vegas. Generally it happens within 48 minutes. The process of vaman starts, when patients vomits all quath, then advice him to drink quatha (decoction) again and vaman vega. After each vega we ask taste in mouth to patient.

When kapha comes out, the taste in mouth is madhur (Sweet). When Pitta comes out taste of mouth is Amla (Sour), Katu, (pungent), titka (bitter) when vata comes out then vaman vega is with noise and bubbles come with vomited kwatha (decoction).

Licked pasted be vomited out. This will be last vega of vaman. Vaman vegas and Type of Shuddhi -

1. Jaghanya - 4 vaman vega
2. Madhay - 6 vaman vega
3. Pravar - 8 vaman vega

Patient is then adviced Dhoompana (smoking) vidhi for remaining shesha dosha by vacha (calamus) churna. (Powder) Smoke of vacha churna inhaled through mouth and nose for 2 to 3 times.

8) POST PROCEDURE (Pashchat) KARMA

1) Patients is adviced to take total rest for 3 to 5 days.

2) Sleeping in day time, maithuna (Sexual activity), ratri jagaran (awakening at night) should be avoided.

3) For 7 days patient should drink warm water.

Special Diet - Sansarjana karma.

1) **Manda** (मंड) (Clear Soup) - 1 bowl - Rice + 16 bowl water are cooked together - then filtere it. Only that processed water should be taken for 1st day.

2) **Peya** (पेया) - (Soup) 1 bowl Rice + 8 bowl water cooked together then filtered. This is for II-Ind day.

3) **Yusha** (यूष) (Semisolid Soup) - (a) Kruta -

processed with herbs, (b) (Akruta) plain rice 1 bowl rice + 8 bowl water cooked together 1/2 rice should be taken.

4) **Vilepi** - 1 part rice + 4 part water cooked together making paste of cooked rice for third day.

This sansarjana karma should be adviced from 3 to 7 days according to the vaman vega shudhi.

9) Thus vaman karma (Emesis) helps to cure E.N.T. - Eye disorders.

Chapter : 28

Clinical trials

The role of Anu Taila nasya in treatment of netra roga (eye diseases)

- Vd. Shailaja R. Kulkarni and
Vd. S. M. Sathye (Pune)

In netra roga Aschyotandi sthanik (local) treatment is common. But to see the effect of nasya, the subject is chosen.

Criteria for selection of patients :

Patients suffering from + (plus) netra roga (refractive error) (Diffuseovision) are selected for study (Total no. 48) and divided in two groups according to age.

Group 1 : 8 to 25 years

Group 2 : 15 to 25 years

Drug Used : Anu Taila

Dose : 1 drop in each nostril at bed time.

Duration : 1½ months.

Follow up : Every eight days (per week)

Observation :

Prakruti	No. of Patients	Percentage
Kaphapradhan	21	52.5%
Vatapradhan	17	42.5%
Pittapradhan	2	5.0%

Male	19	47.5%
Female	21	52.5%
Age 6 to 15	18	45%
16 to 30	22	55%
Upashaya	38	95%
Anupashaya	2	5%

Inference :

In netra roga when kapha-vata dushti is prominent. Anu Taila nasya gives excellent effect.

But vision can not be increased by Anu Taila nasya (At least in the period of two months).

2. The effect of Ghrut Nasya in the management of ardhavbheda (Hemicrania)

Ardhavbheda is a disease comparable to migrain. For this disease in modern medicine has its own limitation. The prolonged use endangers persistant vascular spasm in patient who have vascular disease, similarly the ergot preparations are to be used carefully in case of pregnant women. Ergot has to be given in range of 10 to 15 mg. per week. This does schedule is not free from risk. Even in healthy individuals ergot itself causes headache. Drugs like propanolol produce retroperitoneal fibrosis. This complication is reported in many cases when the patient has been treated continuously for more than 3 to 4 moths.

Considering the above factors an attempt is made to find out an useful Ayurvedic remedy for ardhavbhedak.

Clinical test :

Total no. of patients : 42

5 patients were studied by modern physician. 37 patients were studied by Ayurvedic physician.

Drug :

Goghrita nasya - 2 drops - 3 times (7 a.m., 2 p.m., 9 p.m.)

Nasya chikitsa by this way was given for three months.

Conclusion :

The treatment for ardhavbheda by modern medicine i.e. for migraine is having limited scope and has many side effects and complications.

Simple treatment of ghrita nasya can give relief to a considerable extent.